I0693596

Bodegas

"To the vibrant urban youth who breathe life into our cities: May you recognize the power of choice in every bite and embrace the path to vitality. Let the allure of the Bodega's unhealthy temptations be overshadowed by the promise of a stronger, healthier future. Your well-being is our hope and our legacy."

-Dr. Josh J. Mack

Bodegas:

Urban Children Health Matters

(English Edition)

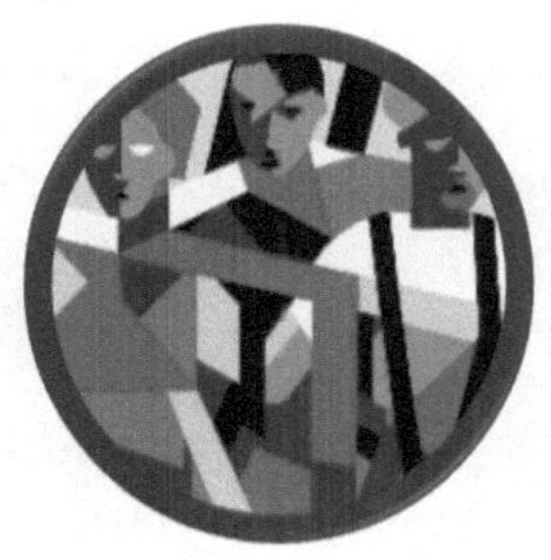

Dr. Josh J. Mack

Kindle Publishing

Copyright © 2023 by Dr. Josh J. Mack. All rights reserved.

No part of this book may be reproduced, stored in a retrieval system, or transmitted in any form or by any means—electronic, mechanical, photocopying, recording, or otherwise—without the prior written permission of the copyright holder.

This book is protected under the copyright laws of United State/New York. Unauthorized reproduction or distribution of this copyrighted work is illegal and may result in severe civil and criminal penalties.

For permissions requests, please contact Dr. Josh J. Mack at www.exceles.org, urbanteacher28@gmail.com, or (585)802-3855.

Any unauthorized copying, distribution, or use of this book, in whole or in part, without permission from the copyright holder is strictly prohibited and may be liable for legal action.

Please note that while every precaution has been taken to ensure the accuracy and reliability of the information presented in this book, the author and publisher shall not be held responsible for any errors or omissions, or for any consequences arising from the use of the information contained herein.

This copyright statement applies to all editions of the book, including electronic or digital formats.

ISBN: 9798333110114 (Paperback)

LCCN: 2023915998

Contents

Acknowledgement

Writing "Bodegas: Urban Children Health Matters" has been an illuminating journey, one that I could not have undertaken without the support, encouragement, and insights of countless individuals. It is with profound gratitude that I acknowledge their invaluable contributions.

Firstly, I must express my deepest appreciation to the Urban children of my community who always welcomed me into their lives, willing to debate me on why they make the food choice they do. Your narratives are the heart and soul of this book. The children, whose health and future this book centers around, have been my driving force.

I am indebted to my mentors, especially Mr. John Norris, Mrs. Beullah Patterson, Mrs. Edna Craven, Mrs. Delaine Cook-Green, and Bishop Herman Daley whose pioneering work in community health and development laid the foundation for this long overdue book. Their wisdom, guidance, and unwavering belief in my vision in years past have been instrumental.

Lastly, I'd like to acknowledge every reader who picks up this book. By seeking to understand, empathize, and act, you are an essential part of the solution. Together, let's champion the health and well-being of Urban children everywhere.

With immense gratitude,

Dr. Josh J. Mack
Dr. Josh J. Mack

About the Author

Dr. Josh J. Mack is not just an educator but a luminary in the realm of community health. With a steadfast commitment to improving the lives of the underserved, his journey began in the classrooms where he imparted knowledge and insights to the next generation. Recognizing the profound connection between education and health, Dr. Mack transitioned into the field of community health advocacy, intent on making a tangible difference.

"Bodegas: Urban Children Health Matters" is an amalgamation of Dr. Mack's years of rigorous research, firsthand experiences, and his intimate understanding of the African American community. Through the pages of this book, he delves deep into the challenges faced by Urban children in urban landscapes, emphasizing the pivotal role bodegas play in shaping their nutritional habits and overall health.

Dr. Mack has often been hailed as a bridge-builder, seamlessly connecting the dots between education, health, culture, and community development. He believes that empowering communities starts with understanding their unique narratives, challenges, and strengths.

When he isn't advocating for better health policies or teaching, Dr. Mack is often found engaging with community leaders, parents, and children, understanding their stories and co-creating solutions. He is a firm believer in the adage, "It takes a village," and through his book, he hopes to inspire that village to rally for the health and future of its youngest members.

Dr. Mack's dedication isn't confined to his professional endeavors. Outside of his advocacy work, he often mentors young educators and health professionals, ensuring that his legacy of care, understanding, and action continues for generations to come.

Introduction

In the bustling streets of urban America, amidst the symphony of car horns, footsteps, and the distant rhythms of city life, stands a silent sentinel: the neighborhood bodega. These corner stores, often unassuming in appearance, hold a potent cultural significance, representing more than just a place to grab a quick snack or household essential. They have become an integral part of urban fabric, offering convenience and a touch of community spirit in the midst of sprawling metropolises. Yet, while they play this key societal role, bodegas have inadvertently become battlegrounds in the fight for better health among Urban children.

"Bodegas: Urban Children Health Matters" delves deep into the complex interplay between these corner stores and the health outcomes of Urban children residing in urban settings. As the subsequent chapters will elucidate, while these stores offer an array of goods, the preponderance of sugary, fatty, and processed foods poses critical challenges. For many Urban families, especially those in underserved neighborhoods, bodegas are sometimes the most accessible — or even the only — food sources available. This availability, juxtaposed with the dearth of fresh, nutritious options, can lead to significant health implications.

This book is not just a critique, but also an exploration. It seeks to unravel the historical, socioeconomic, and cultural threads that have woven the current tapestry of food access in Urban communities. It aims to shed light on the challenges, while also highlighting the potential for positive change, community resilience, and the indomitable spirit that defines these neighborhoods.

Join me on this enlightening journey through the aisles of the local bodega, as I examine their impact, their potential, and the vital importance of ensuring that when it comes to the health of Urban children, every choice matters.

Author's Story

Several years ago, I managed an academic and employment training program for urban youth aged 14 to 21. My organization also collaborated with a local health food provider called FoodLink to offer daily healthy and nutritious hot meals to our participants.

In the program's early weeks, we educated our students about the benefits of a healthy diet and the cost savings of avoiding purchases from bodegas. We encouraged them to choose meals from our health-conscious menu. Initially, we faced resistance; many students persisted in bringing meals from bodegas and fast-food restaurants.

Despite the challenges, our staff demonstrated commitment by consistently choosing FoodLink's meals. As a result, there were often leftovers, which staff could take home for dinner.

However, by the third week, we noticed a shift. More students began choosing our healthy offerings over bodega options. In time, the demand increased so much that there were no leftovers for our staff. We even engaged students in cooking healthy dishes to share with their peers, turning the initiative into a resounding success. The takeaway from this experience is:

"Consistency, leading by example, and patience can influence positive change, even when faced with initial resistance. Over time, persistent efforts can shape healthier choices and behaviors in youth."

-Dr. Josh J. Mack

Chapter 1: Historical Threads of Food Access in Urban Communities

Introduction

Understanding the dynamics of food access in Black communities requires a deep dive into historical contexts. Over the years, systemic factors such as racial discrimination, economic disparities, and urban development have influenced food access for Black Americans. This chapter examines the historical thread that has contributed to the current state of food availability and choice in Urban neighborhoods.

The Legacy of Slavery and Sharecropping

"Throughout American history, Black families have been deeply intertwined with agricultural systems, often being subjected to its harshest conditions, whether as enslaved workers on vast plantations or as sharecroppers in the turbulent post-Civil War era (Dubois, 1935). This agricultural involvement, paradoxically, did not grant them the freedom or autonomy to cultivate crops for their own nourishment.

Often, these families were relegated to consuming the residuals from harvests – the leftover, frequently nutritionally deficient parts that plantation owners deemed unsellable (Kumanyika, 2008).

As Coates (2014) asserts, these systemic oppressions paved the way for broader economic disparities, which, over time, impacted food choices. This history laid the foundation for patterns of food insecurity that weren't merely based on availability but were deeply entrenched in systemic inequities, leading to a significant reliance on less healthy and nourishing food options (Williams, 2006). The evolution of these patterns, when juxtaposed against modern urban development and societal shifts, further underscores the importance of considering the nexus of history, socioeconomic factors, and food choices in Black communities (Gottlieb & Joshi, 2010; White, 2011)."

The Great Migration

"The period between 1916 and 1970 witnessed what historians and scholars refer to as the Great Migration, a significant demographic shift in which millions of Black Americans moved from the rural Southern states to urban centers in the North, West, and Midwest (Coates, 2014). This migration, fueled by a desire for better economic opportunities and escape from racial segregation and Jim Crow laws, also marked a considerable shift from agrarian lifestyles to urban living. Consequently, many Black families found themselves disconnected from direct agricultural and food production practices that they once knew (Kumanyika, 2008).

The transition to urban life meant a reliance on the urban food system. However, this system, even in its nascent stages, was not uniformly distributed or accessible. In many Northern cities, discriminatory policies and systemic racism, not unlike the Southern systems they were escaping, meant that Urban neighborhoods were often underserved with essential amenities, including grocery stores and fresh produce markets (Morland et al., 2002). Such disparities in food access in these areas were, and still are, reflective of broader systemic inequalities that have roots in America's long history of racial discrimination (Dubois, 1935).

This scarcity of nutritious and affordable food options in urban settings laid the groundwork for reliance on less healthy alternatives often found in corner stores or fast-food establishments, which tended to proliferate in such underserved neighborhoods (Powell et al., 2007). The combined effects of being uprooted from direct food production and contending with limited nutritious food choices in urban settings further exacerbated the challenges Black families faced in maintaining a balanced diet and contributed to the widening nutritional health gap (Williams, 2006; Kumanyika, 2008)."

Redlining and Economic Disparities

"In the 1930s, amidst the socio-economic challenges that were already present, the policy of redlining emerged, fundamentally altering the prospects of Black communities in America (Coates, 2014). This racially discriminatory practice, propagated by banks and housing agencies, systematically refused loans or insurance to homeowners in predominantly

Black neighborhoods, labeling them as 'high risk' areas on red-shaded maps (Dubois, 1935). As a direct consequence, economic growth in these neighborhoods was stunted, causing many Black communities to face prolonged economic stagnation and making homeownership, a crucial source of wealth accumulation in America, an elusive dream for many Urban families (Kumanyika, 2008).

The ramifications of redlining extended beyond housing. As neighborhoods were deemed unworthy of financial investments, this sentiment indirectly translated to commercial disinterest. Over time, these areas, already grappling with economic challenges, were bypassed by businesses, further entrenching the divide. Notably, supermarkets and stores offering fresh produce were scarce in these areas, exacerbating the challenges of accessing nutritious food (Morland et al., 2002). The absence of these vital food sources, combined with limited economic resources, fostered environments known today as "food deserts." These zones are characterized by their lack of fresh fruit, vegetables, and other healthful whole foods, and are typically found in impoverished areas due to a lack of grocery stores, farmers' markets, and healthy food providers (Powell et al., 2007).

The food insecurity faced in these neighborhoods, a direct consequence of redlining and economic neglect, is more than just a question of accessibility. It ties into broader narratives of systemic racism, economic discrimination, and health disparities, with residents of these areas facing higher rates of nutrition-related illnesses and conditions (Williams, 2006; Kumanyika, 2008). As scholars and activists address these issues, they underline the significance of food justice, which seeks to ensure that the benefits and risks of where, what, and how food is grown, produced, transported,

distributed, accessed, and eaten are shared fairly (Gottlieb &
Joshi, 2010)."

Emergence of Fast Food and Corner Stores

"In neighborhoods hit hardest by economic stagnation, a
void began to form in the availability of fresh and nutritious
food. Supermarkets and fresh produce vendors, which
traditionally offered a variety of wholesome foods, became a
rarity in these areas. However, this void was soon filled, not
with healthier alternatives, but rather with establishments that
prioritized convenience and cost over nutrition (Powell et al.,
2007). Fast food chains, known for their quick and affordable
meals, rapidly proliferated in these underserved
neighborhoods. Similarly, corner stores, often limited in their
selection, largely stocked processed, sugar-laden, and calorie-
dense products, which, while economical, were nutrient-poor
(Morland et al., 2002).

This shift towards convenience-oriented food outlets
presented immediate and tangible solutions to hunger but
inadvertently created long-term health concerns. For many
African Americans in these neighborhoods, the limited access
to fresh produce and over-reliance on processed foods
contributed to dietary patterns that were high in salt, sugar,
and unhealthy fats (Williams, 2006). This not only widened
the nutritional health gap but also exacerbated the risk of
chronic diseases like obesity, diabetes, and cardiovascular
diseases, which have since been observed to be

disproportionately prevalent in these communities (Kumanyika, 2008).

The omnipresence of these less nutritious food options in Black neighborhoods, coupled with the relative scarcity of healthy alternatives, was more than just an outcome of market forces. It can be seen as an extension of the systemic inequities rooted in policies like redlining and the broader history of racial discrimination. The consequences of these structural determinants manifested not only in the economic fabric of these communities but also in their health outcomes (Kumanyika, 2008; Coates, 2014). As scholars have pointed out, food justice isn't just about access; it's deeply intertwined with broader narratives of social justice, equity, and the right to a healthy life (Gottlieb & Joshi, 2010)."

Urban Renewal Programs

"In the mid-20th century, the landscapes of many American cities were undergoing transformative changes under the banner of 'urban renewal.' Often touted as rejuvenation projects aimed at eliminating urban blight, these initiatives disproportionately targeted neighborhoods with significant Urban populations, reshaping their socio-economic and cultural fabrics (Coates, 2014). Anderson and Christian (2012) highlight that these redevelopment programs often had an underlying intention: the removal or "cleansing" of spaces perceived as deteriorated, which inadvertently were areas with high concentrations of Urban families.

One of the less discussed casualties of these urban renewal programs was the displacement of community-driven local food sources. Community gardens, which had served not just as sources of fresh produce but also as centers of community bonding and cultural preservation, were razed to make way for commercial or upscale residential properties (White, 2011). Such gardens, cultivated often as acts of resilience in the face of food insecurity, were symbols of self-reliance and autonomy. Their loss further exacerbated the already pressing issue of limited access to fresh and healthy food options (Gottlieb & Joshi, 2010).

As these local food sources diminished, the neighborhood residents were thrust further into dependency on external, often less nutritious, food options. The spaces that once bore fruit and vegetables now bore concrete structures, contributing to the rise of "food deserts" — urban zones where fresh, affordable food was hard to come by (Morland et al., 2002). The implications of these urban transformations were manifold: not only did they affect the physical health of the residents due to restricted access to fresh produce (Williams, 2006; Kumanyika, 2008), but they also contributed to the erosion of community spirit and cultural continuity that these gardens symbolized (Reynolds & Cohen, 2016).

In hindsight, while urban renewal projects promised rejuvenation and development, they often stripped Urban neighborhoods of essential cultural, communal, and nutritional resources, leaving behind lasting scars in their wake (Dubois, 1935). The complex interplay of urban development, racial dynamics, and food justice remains a crucial area of study, revealing layers of systemic inequities and their impact on Urban communities."

Economic Barriers

"Across the span of American history, Urban communities have faced significant economic challenges, including disproportionately higher rates of unemployment and underemployment compared to their white counterparts (Coates, 2014). Such disparities have been rooted in systemic racial prejudices and discriminatory policies that have consistently hindered economic mobility within these communities (Dubois, 1935). Anderson and Christian (2012) further emphasize the long-standing economic marginalization faced by Black Americans, suggesting that it has been a pivotal factor contributing to food insecurity in these communities.

Financial constraints inherently influence purchasing decisions. For many Urban families, limited financial resources have necessitated difficult choices in everyday expenses, especially when it comes to food (Williams, 2006). While the ideal choice is fresh and nutritious food, these often come at a premium, rendering them inaccessible to many who are already struggling to make ends meet (Gottlieb & Joshi, 2010).

Such economic constraints, coupled with the absence of easily accessible outlets offering healthy food options in many Urban neighborhoods, exacerbate the problem (Morland et al., 2002; Powell et al., 2007). As a result, cheaper alternatives become the go-to. These alternatives, including fast foods or processed foods available at local corner stores, are typically calorie-dense, offering immediate satiety but are nutritionally poor (Kumanyika, 2008). Consuming such foods over prolonged periods can have detrimental health outcomes, widening the health disparities that already exist due to socio-economic factors (Williams, 2006).

Moreover, initiatives like urban gardening, which sought to counter the scarcity of fresh produce in many Black communities, have faced challenges ranging from displacement due to urban redevelopment to insufficient support and resources (White, 2011; Reynolds & Cohen, 2016). Thus, while the community has shown resilience and ingenuity in trying to address food security issues, systemic barriers continue to pose significant challenges.

In essence, the economic struggles of Black communities, deeply rooted in America's historical and systemic racial biases, have had cascading effects on various aspects of life, notably food choice. The intricate link between economic capability and access to nutritious food requires comprehensive solutions that address not just food distribution but also the underlying socio-economic inequities."

Conclusion

The trajectory of food access in Black communities in the U.S. is an intricate tapestry woven from historical, racial, economic, and socio-political threads. Rooted in America's history is a legacy of systemic racial discrimination that has, in many ways, shaped the socio-economic landscape of Black communities. Deliberate policies, both public and private, have historically disadvantaged Urban Americans, creating a backdrop for contemporary challenges, including food inequity.

One manifestation of these challenges is evident in the choices and decisions Black families often face regarding their nutrition. The economic constraints experienced by many Black families, a consequence of long-standing systemic inequities, mean that purchasing power is often limited. Consequently, when fresh, nutritious food comes at a premium, many are pushed towards more affordable, calorie-dense, but less nutritious options. This is not merely a reflection of personal choice but the result of an environment where healthier options are neither accessible nor affordable.

The spatial dynamics of neighborhoods further illuminate this challenge. Research has shown that Black neighborhoods often lack ready access to stores that stock fresh produce or nutritious food options. Such disparities are not mere coincidences but rather the consequences of long-standing structural and economic decisions that have placed commercial interests over community health.

However, in the face of these challenges, there have been resilient responses from within Black communities. Urban gardening movements, for instance, have emerged as acts of resistance and empowerment against the backdrop of food deserts. Such endeavors, as chronicled in cities like Detroit and New York, represent community-led efforts to reclaim food sovereignty and assert the right to fresh, nutritious food.

In crafting interventions to address food inequities, understanding this intricate history is paramount. Solutions that are not rooted in an understanding of the deep-seated forces that have shaped food access in Black communities are bound to be superficial and short-lived. By acknowledging and addressing these systemic forces, stakeholders—from policymakers to community leaders—can craft more sustainable and impactful interventions, ensuring that equitable food access becomes a realized right for Black communities, not just an aspiration.

Chapter 2: Impact of Corner Stores on Urban Children's Health

Introduction

Neighborhood corner stores, often colloquially known as "bodegas" in some urban settings, play a significant role in the daily lives of many residents, especially in underserved communities. These small-scale retail outlets offer convenience, but their inventory often emphasizes processed, sugary, and fatty foods. For Urban children who may rely on these stores for snacks and even basic groceries, there are concerning health implications.

Limited Access to Nutritious Foods

Corner stores, especially those in urban settings, have a proclivity towards the stocking of non-perishable items, with many often sidelining or even omitting fresh produce entirely (Borradaile et al., 2009). This oversight can lead to significant repercussions on health, especially for children, as the paucity of fruits, vegetables, and whole foods might culminate in nutrient deficiencies (Larson, Story, & Nelson, 2009).

Furthermore, on the rare occasions when fresh produce does find its way into these stores, the prices are usually escalated.

This inflation can be attributed to the limited scale of corner stores, which unlike their larger counterparts, lack the purchasing power to negotiate bulk rates or discounts, consequently passing the added cost onto the consumers (Cummins & Macintyre, 2006; Laska et al., 2010). This economic dimension intensifies the challenge of accessing healthy food options for many families, particularly those in African American communities, where targeted food and beverage marketing plays a significant role in shaping dietary choices (Grier & Kumanyika, 2008; Kumanyika, 2008).

High Availability of Unhealthy Options

Corner stores, especially in urban environments, predominantly showcase a range of high-calorie, low-nutrient foods, including chips, candies, sugary beverages, and processed meat products (Borradaile et al., 2009). The presence of these items, often displayed prominently, can easily trigger impulse purchases, further exacerbating the consumption of unhealthy food items (Borradaile et al., 2009). This dietary pattern, which is influenced by the limited availability of nutritious food in corner stores, poses significant health threats. When consumed routinely, such foods are linked to weight gain, dental issues, and other related health problems, especially among Urban children (Larson, Story, & Nelson, 2009).

The local food environment plays a critical role in shaping dietary choices. For instance, neighborhoods that predominantly have corner stores rather than full-scale grocery outlets can inadvertently promote unhealthy dietary patterns (Cummins & Macintyre, 2006). These patterns are intensified in neighborhoods characterized as "food deserts," where healthy and affordable food choices are scarce (Walker, Keane, & Burke, 2010). Moreover, targeted food and beverage marketing strategies towards African Americans further compound the problem by pushing unhealthy choices to the forefront of consumer awareness (Grier & Kumanyika, 2008). These dynamics converge, creating an environment where ethnic and cultural factors become significant determinants in the rising rates of childhood obesity, especially in Urban communities (Kumanyika, 2008). While the challenges are manifold, addressing them requires a deep understanding of the nuanced interplay between store availability, product placement, pricing, and community demographics (Laska et al., 2010).

Economic Implications and Food Deserts

Many Urban neighborhoods in the U.S. are situated within what researchers' term "food deserts." These are locales characterized by limited access to fresh and nutritious foods, primarily due to the absence of full-service grocery stores (Walker, Keane, & Burke, 2010). Instead, residents of these neighborhoods often find themselves surrounded by corner stores, which typically stock a limited range of perishable goods, focusing more on high-calorie, low-nutrient foods like chips, candies, and sugary beverages (Borradaile et al., 2009).

The layout of food environments, in part, is shaped by broader socioeconomic structures that manifest on a neighborhood scale (Cummins & Macintyre, 2006). For families living in these regions, the economic cost of traveling to distant supermarkets, both in terms of time and money, may outweigh the perceived benefits of purchasing healthier foods. Consequently, many might opt for the more accessible, albeit less nutritious, options available in their local corner stores (Larson, Story, & Nelson, 2009). This decision is further influenced by the targeted food and beverage marketing strategies, which often prioritize products that are less healthy but more profitable, especially towards African American consumers (Grier & Kumanyika, 2008).

Moreover, when juxtaposed with other urban areas, the disparities in healthy food availability become even more pronounced. Studies comparing food store environments across multiple U.S. cities have highlighted the significant variability in the presence of healthy foods, with some cities having corner stores that offer markedly fewer nutritious options (Laska et al., 2010). These urban environments, coupled with cultural and ethnic influences, contribute to the broader environmental factors affecting childhood obesity, especially among Urban children (Kumanyika, 2008). As a result, a deeper understanding of both the micro and macro-level dynamics at play is essential for devising strategies that promote better food choices and health outcomes for these communities.

Cultural and Social Factors

Peer pressure and prevailing societal norms play significant roles in shaping individual food choices, especially among children. The local food environment often mirrors these societal influences. For instance, corner stores, which are frequently found in urban neighborhoods, predominantly stock high-calorie, low-nutrient items (Borradaile et al., 2009). Such stores, which are positioned as convenient go-to places, tend to prominently display snack foods, potentially triggering impulse purchases (Borradaile et al., 2009).

Within the African American community, targeted food and beverage marketing strategies have particularly emphasized these less nutritious products, fostering a sense of normalization around their consumption (Grier & Kumanyika, 2008). This targeted approach can make it challenging for individuals, especially children, to make healthier food choices even when they are available (Laska et al., 2010). The widespread availability of such foods in neighborhood stores thus provides a backdrop against which peer interactions occur.

When children see their peers frequently purchasing and consuming these unhealthy snacks, they are likely to perceive such behaviors as standard. This perception can create a loop where the behavior is continually reinforced, leading to a community-wide acceptance of such dietary habits (Kumanyika, 2008). For Urban children, especially those residing in neighborhoods categorized as "food deserts" with limited access to healthy foods, this cyclical pattern presents a heightened risk. The restricted availability of fresh and nutritious foods coupled with the prominence of unhealthy options in local stores makes them more susceptible to adopting these detrimental dietary habits (Walker, Keane, & Burke, 2010; Larson, Story, & Nelson, 2009).

Therefore, understanding the interplay between the physical food environment, targeted marketing strategies, and societal norms is crucial when considering the dietary behaviors of Urban children and the broader implications for their health (Cummins & Macintyre, 2006).

Long-term Health Concerns

Childhood is a critical period for the establishment of dietary habits, which, once ingrained, can prove difficult to modify later in life (Kumanyika, 2008). The local food environment plays a pivotal role in shaping these habits. Notably, in several urban settings, corner stores have become staples in neighborhoods, offering residents, including children, a convenient place to purchase food items (Borradaile et al., 2009). However, the foods prominently displayed in such stores tend to be high-calorie, low-nutrient products that can stimulate impulse purchases, further reinforcing the normalization of processed food consumption (Borradaile et al., 2009; Laska et al., 2010).

The implications of a diet dominated by processed foods are far-reaching. For Urban children, an early and consistent exposure to such foods elevates their risk for chronic health conditions like obesity, diabetes, heart disease, and hypertension in the future (Kumanyika, 2008). Regrettably, these health conditions already show a disproportionate prevalence within the Urban community, in part due to systemic issues like disparities in access to fresh, healthy foods and the prominence of food deserts (Walker, Keane, & Burke, 2010; Larson, Story, & Nelson, 2009).

Furthermore, targeted marketing campaigns have further exacerbated this issue. The African American community, including its youngest members, is often the target of food and beverage marketing that emphasizes less nutritious options (Grier & Kumanyika, 2008). Such targeted strategies, paired with limited healthy food options in neighborhoods, make it challenging for Urban children to routinely make healthy dietary choices (Cummins & Macintyre, 2006).

In sum, the interplay of local food environments, marketing strategies, and broader systemic issues lays the groundwork for dietary habits that, if unchecked, can predispose Urban children to a host of chronic health challenges that persist into adulthood (Kumanyika, 2008).

Potential for Positive Change

The food environment in neighborhoods has been identified as a significant factor influencing dietary habits, particularly in urban areas where corner stores play a pivotal role in residents' daily food purchases (Borradaile et al., 2009). Notably, many of these corner stores predominantly stock unhealthy, high-calorie snacks and drinks, which can facilitate impulse purchases and contribute to poor dietary habits (Borradaile et al., 2009). In light of these challenges, several initiatives have been put forward to reshape the food landscape in these areas.

One proactive approach has involved collaborations with corner store owners to modify the availability of food options within their stores. Specifically, these collaborations aim to increase the stock of healthier food choices and reduce the prominence of unhealthy snacks and beverages that contribute to negative health outcomes (Laska et al., 2010). By transforming the physical food environment within these stores, the hope is to make nutritious options more accessible and appealing to the community, potentially influencing purchasing behaviors (Larson, Story, & Nelson, 2009).

Beyond physical changes to the food environment, there's also a significant role for education and community outreach. Informing both parents and children about the importance of nutritious food choices can empower individuals to make healthier decisions, even when faced with less-than-optimal food environments (Cummins & Macintyre, 2006). These educational efforts are particularly crucial in communities targeted by food and beverage marketing that emphasizes less healthy options (Grier & Kumanyika, 2008). By creating an informed community, the potential for collective behavior change grows, leading to a shift in dietary norms and practices.

Moreover, understanding the broader societal and cultural contexts, especially as they relate to childhood obesity in different ethnic groups, can help tailor these educational efforts more effectively (Kumanyika, 2008). By approaching the issue of unhealthy food environments holistically, combining both store-level interventions and community education, there's an increased chance of creating lasting positive change in communities' dietary habits and overall health.

Conclusion

Neighborhood corner stores, often situated within walking distance for many urban residents, have become integral fixtures in daily life, especially for those who might not have easy access to larger supermarkets or grocery stores. For many Urban communities located in "food deserts," these corner stores frequently serve as primary sources of food due to a lack of alternative options.

However, the convenience offered by these stores can be overshadowed by the nutritional challenges they present. Research has revealed that these corner stores typically have a plethora of high-calorie, processed snacks and beverages, often displayed in ways that trigger impulse purchases. This prominence of unhealthy options can inadvertently guide purchasing behaviors, especially among children who may lack the knowledge or experience to make health-conscious decisions.

Given this context, Urban children who rely on corner stores for daily nutrition are exposed to a disproportionate risk of adopting unhealthy dietary habits. This situation is further exacerbated by targeted food and beverage marketing strategies directed towards African Americans, which emphasize calorie-dense, nutrient-poor options. Over time, consistent exposure to such an environment can predispose Urban children to a range of chronic health conditions, including obesity and its associated complications, conditions that are already prevalent in the Urban community.

Thus, understanding the nuanced relationships between corner store environments, targeted marketing, and health outcomes becomes paramount for those interested in safeguarding the well-being of Urban communities. Policymakers, community leaders, and parents all have roles to play. For instance, initiatives like partnering with store owners to enhance the availability of healthier options are steps in the right direction.

As community stakeholders work towards creating healthier food environments, the combined effort can potentially shift dietary norms, fostering a community where convenience does not come at the cost of health.

Chapter 3: High-Calorie Foods & Physical Health in Urban Children

Introduction

In the United States, Urban children grapple with a myriad of health disparities. These disparities arise from a nuanced matrix of socioeconomic, environmental, and cultural dynamics. A salient concern echoing across Urban communities is the omnipresence of high calorie, low nutritional value foods. This concern is particularly magnified within regions recognized as "food deserts," where avenues to acquire fresh, healthy food are conspicuously sparse. This chapter sheds light on the repercussions of such dietary patterns on Urban children's health.

The Nutritional Paradox

The pervasive presence of high-calorie, low-nutrient foods in many communities creates a challenging paradox. These foods, often loaded with sugars, trans fats, and salt, offer a deceptive bounty—abundant in calories but deficient in essential nutrients (Borradaile et al., 2009). As a result, even as children consume more than enough energy, they miss out on the vital vitamins, minerals, and other necessary nutrients crucial for their growth, cognitive development, and overall health. This situation is not merely a matter of individual choices but is deeply embedded in the larger food environment.

In urban areas, particularly, the ease of access to such nutrient-deficient foods is evident. Corner stores in cities like Philadelphia prominently display snack foods that might trigger impulse purchases, thereby increasing the chances of children consuming these high calorie yet nutritionally poor products (Borradaile et al., 2009). Moreover, certain neighborhoods in the U.S. have notable disparities in their access to healthier food alternatives (Larson, Story, & Nelson, 2009). This environment, marked by a dearth of nutritious options and an excess of unhealthy ones, positions children in a challenging spot nutritionally.

However, it's not just about accessibility; it's also about influence. Targeted marketing strategies often propel these high-calorie foods to the forefront for African American communities (Grier & Kumanyika, 2008). The cultural and environmental contexts further accentuate these patterns, adding layers of complexity to the issue of childhood obesity and malnutrition within these communities (Kumanyika, 2008).

Cummins & Macintyre (2006) emphasized the broader implications of such food environments on obesity, suggesting that the problems may lie at the level of neighborhoods or even nations. This brings forth a stark realization: children might be overfed in terms of calories but undernourished when it comes to essential nutrients—a dilemma that requires comprehensive strategies for resolution. Solutions may lie in initiatives like diversifying food availability in urban stores across different cities, as highlighted by Laska et al. (2010), or addressing the broader disparities in food access (Walker, Keane, & Burke, 2010).

Health Implications

The pervasive consumption of high-calorie, nutrient-poor foods has profoundly and adversely affected Urban children's health outcomes. With these unhealthy dietary habits becoming more ingrained, there has been a discernible surge in obesity rates among Urban children—a connection emphatically highlighted by Kumanyika (2008). This rise in obesity is not merely a cosmetic concern; it has serious health implications.

Obesity, especially during childhood, significantly increases the risk of developing a spectrum of chronic health conditions. Urban children, already at an elevated risk due to the historical and systemic health disparities affecting their community, now find themselves more predisposed to conditions like type 2 diabetes, hypertension, and heart disease (Grier & Kumanyika, 2008). These are conditions that, sadly, are all too familiar to the Urban community. This places an additional burden on a demographic already grappling with a multitude of health challenges.

Beyond the immediate and apparent physical health repercussions, the deficit of essential nutrients in their diets introduces another layer of complications. Proper nutrition plays a foundational role in a child's developmental trajectory. The absence of critical nutrients doesn't only jeopardize physical growth but can also hinder cognitive development, potentially limiting a child's academic and, subsequently, professional potential. Larson, Story, & Nelson (2009) shed light on this very aspect, underlining the importance of a balanced diet for holistic child development.

This combination of factors presents a dire situation, emphasizing the urgency for comprehensive interventions. Efforts to ameliorate the situation range from improving the availability of healthy foods in urban settings (Laska et al., 2010) to addressing the systemic issues that make unhealthy foods more accessible and appealing, especially in areas identified as food deserts (Walker, Keane, & Burke, 2010). The challenge is complex, rooted in a mix of historical, societal, and economic factors, but acknowledging these multifaceted issues is the first step towards forging a path to better health outcomes.

Socio-Cultural Impact

The intricate web of socio-cultural factors influencing dietary choices in Urban communities underscores the depth of the challenge. Central to this concern is the strategic approach taken by food and beverage corporations. It is observed that they disproportionately target Urban communities with aggressive marketing campaigns promoting less nutritious, high-calorie foods and beverages (Grier & Kumanyika, 2008). Such targeted advertising not only perpetuates but exacerbates the consumption of these unhealthy items. This strategy, insidiously effective, embeds these dietary patterns further into the community, making them appear more as a cultural norm rather than a health concern.

Beyond corporate strategies, cultural narratives and community dynamics play a substantial role in shaping food choices. Within Urban communities, certain dietary patterns have become so interwoven with cultural identity and social interactions that they are viewed as norms. Borradaile et al. (2009) highlighted how corner stores in urban environments like Philadelphia prominently display snack foods, potentially triggering impulse purchases. This prevalence and easy accessibility of high-calorie snacks in local stores can inadvertently cement their place in daily consumption routines.

Furthermore, the weight of societal norms and peer influences, especially in areas saturated with these food choices, can further normalize such eating habits. When children witness their peers and family members regularly consuming these items, the behavior is reinforced, making it seem like an acceptable and regular part of their diet. Kumanyika (2008) provided insights into how these environmental and cultural influences converge, shaping childhood obesity trends, especially within ethnic contexts.

The implications are far-reaching. Beyond the immediate health concerns, these patterns affect how Urban children perceive food, health, and their own identities. The pressing need is to disentangle these complex socio-cultural threads to pave the way for healthier futures, requiring holistic approaches that address both the external influences and the internal community dynamics (Larson, Story, & Nelson, 2009).

Recommendations

Addressing the deep-seated dietary challenges in Urban communities necessitates multi-pronged interventions, each tailored to tackle a specific aspect of the problem.

At the individual and community levels, educating families is paramount. Promoting informed dietary choices is a significant step towards countering the influx of high-calorie, low-nutrition foods. Awareness campaigns can play a pivotal role in enlightening both parents and children about the long-term implications of their food choices. Through such drives, they can be empowered to navigate and make healthier decisions even within environments riddled with less nutritious options. Larson, Story, & Nelson (2009) affirm the transformative potential of these awareness initiatives, highlighting how informed choices can mitigate the adverse health impacts arising from an environment replete with unhealthy food temptations.

Dovetailing these efforts should be policy interventions designed to reshape the very environment in which these dietary choices are made. Corner stores, often the lifeline of urban neighborhoods, have a profound influence on the dietary patterns of their patrons. By incentivizing these stores to carry healthier food options, there's an opportunity to subtly shift community preferences towards nutritionally dense foods. Concurrently, regulations can be instated to limit the conspicuous placement and promotion of unhealthy snack foods. Laska et al. (2010) emphasize the efficacy of such policy maneuvers, illustrating how they can act as catalysts in transforming the food landscape of urban neighborhoods.

Lastly, a holistic approach requires the integration of various community stakeholders. By forging collaborations between community leaders, parents, schools, and healthcare professionals, a cohesive strategy can be crafted. This united front ensures that children not only receive consistent messaging about healthy dietary practices but also have access to the necessary resources and support structures that foster these habits. The emphasis, as Grier & Kumanyika (2008) note, should be on creating a context where making healthier choices becomes not just viable but the norm.

In summary, while the challenges are manifold, a concerted, strategic effort drawing on insights from research and community needs can steer the trajectory towards improved health outcomes for Urban children.

Conclusion

The health and well-being of Urban children is increasingly coming under threat, principally due to their exposure to foods that, while calorically abundant, are grievously deficient in essential nutrients. This predicament, however, isn't just the product of individual choices, but rather an intricate web of socio-environmental and commercial factors that collectively mold dietary behaviors.

One significant challenge is the prominent accessibility of unhealthy foods, especially in urban settings. Snack food displays in Philadelphia corner stores, often brimming with high-calorie, low-nutrient items, can lure individuals into impulsive purchases. These stores become inadvertent agents of unhealthy dietary behaviors, not necessarily out of malice, but often due to market dynamics and consumer demand.

Beyond mere availability, the broader food environment plays an instrumental role in shaping dietary choices. The realm of food environments, from neighborhood grocery stores to national food supply chains, can significantly sway obesity trends. The intricate interplay of food availability, pricing, and marketing in these environments can dictate consumption patterns, often to the detriment of vulnerable populations like Urban children.

Adding another layer of complexity is the targeted advertising by food and beverage giants. The disproportionate targeting of Urban communities by these companies further entrenches unhealthy dietary norms within these communities. Such focused marketing not only capitalizes on cultural motifs but also reinforces them, creating a self-sustaining loop of unhealthy consumption.

However, it isn't just about what's available and advertised. The very places children grow up in can facilitate or obstruct access to healthier food alternatives. The disparities in access to wholesome foods across U.S. neighborhoods is evident. These "food deserts" are areas where fresh, nutritious foods are elusive, further complicating the challenge.

These multifaceted influences aren't merely passive backgrounds against which individual choices are made. They actively shape perceptions, preferences, and practices related to food. Environmental factors, especially those embedded in ethnic and cultural contexts, can impact childhood obesity trends.

Navigating this convoluted scenario requires a comprehensive understanding of these determinants. Solutions might lie in reshaping the very food landscapes of urban neighborhoods. By bolstering the availability of nutritious foods in small urban food stores, one can start recalibrating community preferences towards healthier choices.

In essence, while the plight of Urban children's nutrition seems grim, an informed, multifaceted approach can pave the way for a brighter, healthier future for these children.

Chapter 4: High-Calorie Foods & Mental Health in Urban Children

Introduction

Urban children in the United States navigate through a myriad of health disparities influenced by socioeconomic, environmental, and cultural factors. Among these, the access and consumption of high-calorie, low-nutritional foods in many Urban communities stand out prominently. The consequences of this are not limited to physical health. Recent studies indicate a profound impact on the mental well-being of children. This chapter will explore the intricate relationship between such dietary habits and their mental health ramifications for Urban children.

Mental Health Implications

It's indeed distressing that many foods readily available in our neighborhoods, especially those packed with sugars, trans fats, and salts, are calorically dense but nutritionally barren. While they might satiate immediate hunger, they fall woefully short of supplying the essential nutrients vital for brain health and function (Larson, Story, & Nelson, 2009). The correlation between diet and cognitive health becomes more pronounced in children, where consistent consumption of such foods can stifle their cognitive growth and development.

Moreover, the relationship between diet and mental health is an emerging area of concern. Research has shown that excessive consumption of sugars and processed foods can increase the risk of mood disorders in young people. A diet replete with sugar and processed foods is not just a precursor to physical ailments, but also to mental health conditions such as depression and anxiety. This is especially troubling given that the youth are at a critical developmental stage where such disorders can have lasting implications on their overall well-being.

Further complicating the issue is the aggressive marketing of these unhealthy foods, particularly in Urban communities, which skews dietary habits from an early age (Grier & Kumanyika, 2008). And it's not just mental health that's at stake. There's growing evidence to suggest that diets deficient in essential nutrients might contribute to or exacerbate behavioral issues in children.

Conditions like Attention Deficit Hyperactivity Disorder (ADHD), which already pose significant challenges for affected children and their families, may be influenced by dietary factors, adding another layer of complexity to our understanding of the intricate relationship between diet and health. While a direct causative link between high-calorie, low-nutrition foods and suicide rates in Urban children is yet to be unequivocally established, preliminary studies suggest a significant association. Clark et al. (2019) found that among Urban adolescents, those with poor dietary patterns exhibited higher rates of depression and suicidal ideation than their counterparts with healthier diets.

Additionally, the broader environment plays a significant role in shaping dietary choices. A study by Borradaile et al. (2009) highlighted the prominence of impulse-triggering snack foods in Philadelphia corner stores, suggesting an environment that encourages unhealthy food choices. Similar trends have been observed in other urban settings, where the availability of healthy food options is often dwarfed by an array of unhealthy alternatives (Laska et al., 2010).

In light of this, it becomes evident that there is a pressing need to address the broader food environments (Cummins & Macintyre, 2006), especially in areas identified as "food deserts" where access to nutritious foods is limited (Walker, Keane, & Burke, 2010). Ensuring that children have access to and are educated about healthier dietary choices is paramount to their cognitive, mental, and overall health.

Socio-Cultural Impact

Certainly, the complex interplay between food choices and societal structures cannot be overlooked. The marketing landscape and its evident disparities have profound implications on dietary habits. Urban communities, as highlighted by Grier & Kumanyika (2008), face a disproportionate barrage of advertisements for unhealthy food and beverage options. Such targeted marketing not only influences individual food choices but also, over time, molds a community's collective palate and perception of what is 'normal' or 'acceptable' to eat. This insidious effect can foster a food environment that consistently promotes and rewards unhealthy dietary habits.

Moreover, these targeted advertising strategies serve as a reflection of broader systemic inequities. When high-calorie, nutrient-poor foods are not only more available but also more vigorously promoted within specific communities, it sets up a cyclical pattern of consumption that can be challenging to break (Larson, Story, & Nelson, 2009). Over time, this cyclical pattern embeds itself as a societal norm, further entrenching the perceived 'desirability' of these foods, especially among impressionable younger generations.

The societal norms shaped by such environments can also wield significant psychological power. As Kumanyika (2008) postulates, in areas where the intake of high-calorie and low-nutrient foods has become normalized, children who grow up in such settings might face an intensified peer pressure to conform to these dietary standards. This not only influences their immediate food choices but can also play a role in shaping their mental self-perception. When everyone around them is making similar food choices, it becomes challenging for children to perceive their dietary habits as anything but standard, even if these habits might be detrimental to their health.

Furthermore, the constant exposure to these societal norms and peer pressures can have cascading effects on a child's psychological well-being. When children's diets are at odds with what is portrayed as 'ideal' or 'aspirational' in mainstream media, yet concurrently aligned with the prevalent consumption patterns in their immediate surroundings, it can create a conflict in their self-esteem and overall sense of self-worth. Over time, such dissonance can lead to deeper psychological struggles, further underscoring the importance of addressing the broader societal influences on dietary habits.

Recommendations

Promoting positive change in dietary behaviors and their associated mental health outcomes, especially within underserved communities, indeed requires a comprehensive approach. A significant part of this change begins with education. Informative programs can elucidate the intricate relationship between dietary choices and cognitive well-being. Understanding that food environments in certain neighborhoods are plagued by the availability of high-calorie, low-nutrient foods (Borradaile et al., 2009) makes these educational initiatives even more critical **(see Appendix A)**. By instilling knowledge about the mental health implications of food choices, children and parents can be empowered to make decisions that foster both physical and psychological well-being.

However, education alone might not suffice when the environment itself doesn't support healthier choices. This is where policy intervention becomes invaluable. Policymakers, cognizant of the disparities in access to nutritious foods in many U.S. neighborhoods (Larson, Story, & Nelson, 2009), can take cues from findings such as those presented by Laska et al. (2010). For example, they could introduce incentives for store owners to diversify their product range, including more nutrient-rich food options. Such policies can reshape the very food environment that Cummins & Macintyre (2006) discuss, making it conducive for residents to make healthier choices.

Moreover, bolstering community-led initiatives can also play a transformative role. Encouraging community gardening, for instance, not only ensures access to fresh produce but also fosters a sense of community ownership and education around nutrition. These gardens can act as buffers against the proliferation of food deserts, areas that lack access to fresh, healthy, and affordable foods (Walker, Keane, & Burke, 2010).

Furthermore, addressing the potential mental health ramifications stemming from poor dietary habits requires proactive measures. Routine mental health screenings in educational institutions and community centers can be invaluable. Such screenings can facilitate the early identification of children at risk, ensuring timely interventions. This is especially important considering the complex interplay of environmental factors, like targeted food advertising (Grier & Kumanyika, 2008), and their potential impact on the mental well-being of children. By taking a holistic approach that amalgamates education, policy intervention, and proactive mental health initiatives, it becomes feasible to pave the way for healthier communities.

Conclusion

The prevalence of high-calorie, low-nutritional foods, especially within Urban communities, is deeply intertwined with a multitude of challenges extending beyond just physical health implications. One of the underlying factors is the pervasive availability of such foods in these communities. For instance, the pronounced visibility of snack food displays in urban corner stores might foster impulse purchases of these unhealthy options. This easy accessibility, paired with aggressive targeted marketing strategies directed towards African Americans, exacerbates the consumption of these foods.

Yet, the ramifications of such dietary habits transcend the realm of physical health, casting a profound shadow on the mental well-being of Urban children. The broader neighborhood environments play a pivotal role in this regard. Many Urban communities face stark disparities in access to healthy foods. This inequitable food environment, often referred to as 'food deserts,' puts children in a position where their primary food choices are calorically dense but nutritionally deficient. Such dietary patterns not only expose them to physical health risks but also potentially jeopardize their cognitive and emotional development.

Adding to the complexity is the influence of cultural and environmental contexts on childhood obesity. The profound cultural ties and traditions often shape dietary habits, which when coupled with an environment laden with unhealthy food options, can further heighten the risk. Given these multifaceted challenges, solutions cannot be monolithic. For instance, increasing the availability of healthy foods in small urban food stores across various cities could be a promising strategy to alter the existing food landscape.

Recognizing the depth and breadth of this issue is indeed the inaugural step. Only with a comprehensive understanding can we chart a course towards a future where Urban children are not merely physically healthy but are also in an environment that nurtures their mental and emotional well-being.

Chapter 5: Nutrition's Role in Urban Children's Academic Performance

Introduction

Urban children in the United States grapple with various challenges impacting their academic performance. A prominent challenge is the widespread consumption of high-calorie, low-nutritional value foods within their communities. Though the health implications of these foods are well-known, there's growing attention on their potential to hinder academic achievements. This chapter sheds light on the interplay between these dietary choices and the academic outcomes of Urban children.

Implications for Academic Performance

Dietary patterns and choices play an indispensable role in shaping the cognitive trajectory of children. Essential nutrients are foundational pillars for optimal brain function and cognitive health. Regrettably, the lack of these vital nutrients, especially in diets replete with sugars, trans fats, and salts, has been documented to impede cognitive processes crucial for learning and memory (Larson, Story, & Nelson, 2009). These diets, predominant in areas described as "food deserts," are characterized by limited access to fresh and wholesome foods but are saturated with processed items, often available in local corner stores (Walker, Keane, & Burke, 2010; Laska et al., 2010).

The detrimental impacts of such diets extend beyond just cognitive hindrance. High sugar diets, as indicated by research, are known to cause unstable blood sugar levels. This instability can be a significant impediment to a child's attention span, subsequently hampering their ability to focus and engage productively in classroom activities (Cummins & Macintyre, 2006). Such dietary patterns can, over time, compromise the body's immune system, rendering children more susceptible to a range of illnesses. The consequential frequent absences from school due to illness result in missed educational opportunities, placing these children at a disadvantage compared to their peers.

Furthermore, it's essential to consider the broader landscape in which these dietary habits are entrenched. Targeted advertising campaigns by food corporations disproportionately expose Urban communities to unhealthy food choices (Grier & Kumanyika, 2008). Coupled with cultural and societal norms, these marketing strategies have amplified the acceptance and consumption of high-calorie, low-nutritional foods, further embedding these consumption patterns into the community's fabric (Kumanyika, 2008). The combined effect of these dietary choices on cognitive function, attention span, and school attendance underscores the pressing need for interventions at both the community and policy levels.

Socio-Cultural Factors

The intricate dynamics of food marketing, especially in the context of its environment and targeted communities, bear substantial consequences beyond just influencing eating habits. In particular, Urban communities are often the focal points of aggressive marketing campaigns that push unhealthy food choices (Grier & Kumanyika, 2008). This targeted advertising not only instills and perpetuates poor dietary behaviors but can also inadvertently undermine academic performance. By promoting consumption patterns that are antithetical to cognitive well-being, these marketing strategies may erode the academic potentials of Urban children (Larson, Story, & Nelson, 2009).

The environment within which these children live further complicates matters. Many Urban communities are situated in "food deserts," characterized by limited access to fresh, nutritious food options, yet an overabundance of processed, high-calorie, low-nutritional alternatives (Walker, Keane, & Burke, 2010; Larson, Story, & Nelson, 2009). In such settings, corner stores become the primary food sources, often stocking products that cater to impulse purchases triggered by unhealthy snack food displays (Borradaile et al., 2009). This environment, marked by limited healthy food options, becomes a breeding ground for normalized unhealthy dietary habits.

Moreover, the established norms within these communities further reinforce the consumption of high-calorie, low-nutrient foods. As Kumanyika (2008) has highlighted, these prevailing norms can exert a powerful influence over individual dietary behaviors, acting as both a direct and indirect driver of food choices. The communal acceptance and frequent consumption of these foods can amplify peer pressure, affecting the dietary habits of Urban children. Over time, this convergence of targeted advertising, environmental constraints, and community pressures doesn't just determine what's on the plate; it has profound implications on academic habits, cognitive development, and the overall trajectory of these children's lives (Kumanyika, 2008; Cummins & Macintyre, 2006).

Recommendations

Nutrition's influence on cognitive and academic performance cannot be understated, and it's crucial for both schools and local communities to take proactive steps in addressing the prevailing challenges in this domain. Given the disparities in access to healthy foods within many U.S. neighborhoods, particularly in those predominantly inhabited by Urban communities (Larson, Story, & Nelson, 2009; Walker, Keane, & Burke, 2010), targeted interventions are paramount.

Educational programs within schools that emphasize the intricate link between diet and academic performance can serve as invaluable platforms for change. By illuminating the profound effects of dietary choices on cognitive function, these initiatives can empower children and their families to make informed, health-conscious decisions. This is particularly critical in light of the aggressive marketing strategies targeting African American communities, which have been shown to influence dietary behaviors detrimentally (Grier & Kumanyika, 2008).

From a legislative standpoint, policymakers have a unique role in shaping the food landscape. Encouraging healthier food options, especially in urban corner stores known for their impulse-triggering snack food displays (Borradaile et al., 2009), is vital. As Laska et al. (2010) discuss, strategic policy measures such as tax incentives for retailers stocking healthier food options or subsidizing school meal programs with a nutritional focus can make a significant difference. These policy interventions can serve dual purposes: combating the prevalent obesity trends influenced by food environments (Cummins & Macintyre, 2006) and fostering a conducive environment for academic excellence.

Moreover, grassroots community initiatives can further bridge the gap in healthy food accessibility. Community gardens, for instance, not only provide fresh produce but also foster a sense of community ownership and understanding of nutrition (Kumanyika, 2008). Farm-to-school programs, meanwhile, can ensure that children receive fresh, locally sourced, and nutritionally rich meals, subsequently bolstering their cognitive abilities and academic outcomes.

In summary, a multi-pronged approach encompassing education, policy changes, and community-led interventions is imperative to reshape the food environments of Urban children and unlock their full academic potential.

Conclusion

The academic potential of Urban children, like all children, is boundless. However, external factors, including the nutritional landscape they navigate, can play a pivotal role in determining their academic success. The presence of high-calorie, low-nutritional foods in many urban neighborhoods, particularly those predominantly inhabited by Urban families, presents a significant challenge.

One factor exacerbating this issue is the availability of unhealthy food choices in urban settings. For instance, many corner stores in Philadelphia prominently display snack foods that trigger impulse purchases, further encouraging the consumption of nutritionally deficient foods. These food environments, influenced by strategic product placement and aggressive marketing, can be detrimental, not only for physical health but also for cognitive development and, consequently, academic performance.

Furthermore, it's not just about the foods that are available but also about the foods that are not. Numerous studies have shown that there exist stark disparities in access to fresh, healthy foods in many U.S. neighborhoods. These areas, often termed "food deserts," are marked by limited access to supermarkets or vendors selling fresh produce, instead dominated by outlets selling processed, high-calorie foods. The implications of this are two-fold: an increased risk of obesity and related health issues, and potential hindrances to cognitive development and academic achievement due to poor nutrition.

The cultural and environmental backdrop further complicates matters. Ethnic and cultural norms can sometimes inadvertently perpetuate the consumption of high-calorie, low-nutrient foods, with children being especially susceptible to such influences. Moreover, even in places where there are attempts to provide healthier options, disparities persist.

To unlock the immense academic potential of Urban children, it is essential to recognize these challenges and proactively address the barriers. Creating an environment that both provides access to nutritious foods and educates on the importance of a balanced diet is a foundational step towards ensuring that these children have every opportunity to thrive academically and secure a prosperous future.

Chapter 6: Urban Youth Access to Bodega Alcohol & Cigarettes

Introduction

The health and societal implications of underage consumption of cigarettes and alcohol are well-understood and widely acknowledged. However, for Urban youth, the challenges of accessing these substances in neighborhood bodegas pose a significant concern. There are multiple factors, as highlighted in several studies, that contribute to this problem.

Alcohol & Cigarette Marketing Receptivity

Adolescents' receptivity to alcohol marketing is not only indicative of their consumption patterns but acts as a significant gateway towards the initiation of alcohol use. Henriksen et al. (2010) underscored this relationship, emphasizing how young individuals, when continuously exposed to such marketing tactics, become more inclined to start drinking. This inclination is further exacerbated by the tactics employed by tobacco and alcohol marketers at points of sale, notably neighborhood bodegas.

Bodegas, given their proximity to residences and their informal nature, often become primary shopping destinations for adolescents. Henriksen and colleagues (2004) provided a concerning insight into this, noting that cigarette marketing is considerably more prevalent in stores that adolescents frequently visit. Such targeted marketing not only influences the purchasing decisions of these young individuals but also shapes their perception of the products. It's an illustrative example of how exposure to targeted marketing can normalize the consumption of harmful products, leading to early adoption among adolescents (Feighery et al., 2006).

The positioning of these bodegas further adds to the problem. McCarthy et al. (2009) highlighted the correlation between the density of tobacco retailers near schools and an increased incidence of tobacco use among students. The convenience offered by these bodegas, combined with their lax checking systems, facilitates easier access to these harmful products for underaged consumers.

Moreover, when enforcement of underage tobacco laws remains inadequate, these establishments often sell cigarettes without thorough ID checks. Lipperman-Kreda et al. (2016) expounded on this, linking the high density of tobacco outlets and lax ID checks to youths' cigarette smoking behaviors and their beliefs regarding the acceptability of underage smoking. In essence, when young individuals perceive that it's relatively easy to purchase these products without hindrance, it not only influences their consumption patterns but also shapes their beliefs on the acceptability of underage smoking.

In summation, the intricate web of aggressive marketing, ease of accessibility, and poor enforcement around neighborhood bodegas makes them potential hotspots for underaged alcohol and tobacco consumption. Addressing this requires a multidimensional approach, encompassing stricter regulations on marketing, the strategic positioning of such retailers, and stringent enforcement of age restrictions.

Recommendations

Addressing the issue of Urban youth access to alcohol and cigarettes in neighborhood bodegas requires a comprehensive, multi-pronged approach. Here are some recommendations:

1. **Stricter Regulatory Enforcement:**
   - Introduce stiffer penalties for retailers found selling tobacco and alcohol to minors.
   - Increase the frequency of undercover operations and random checks on bodegas and retailers.
   - Implement more rigorous training for store employees on verifying IDs.

2. **Educational Programs:**
   - Schools should introduce or enhance curricula that educate students on the dangers of underage drinking and smoking.
   - Bodegas and other retailers can be mandated to fund or support community-based educational programs that focus on the harms of underage tobacco and alcohol use.

3. **Limit Advertising and Display:**
   - Restrict the placement of tobacco and alcohol advertisements to areas within the store that are less visible to the youth.
   - Prohibit promotions and discounts on tobacco and alcohol products that can appeal to the younger demographic.

4. **Zoning Laws and Licensing:**
   - Limit the number of licenses issued for selling tobacco and alcohol products in areas densely populated with schools.
   - Enforce buffer zones, which would require tobacco and alcohol retailers to be situated a certain distance away from schools, playgrounds, and other youth-centric areas.

5. **Community Engagement:**
   - Engage community leaders and residents in awareness campaigns highlighting the risks associated with underage drinking and smoking.
   - Promote community reporting. Residents can be encouraged to report stores that violate age-restriction rules.

6. **Support for Alternatives:**
   - Offer incentives for bodegas to stock and promote healthier product alternatives.
   - Encourage bodegas to partner with local health initiatives, providing space for health promotion activities or campaigns.

7. **Youth Engagement:**
   - Establish youth advocacy groups that champion anti-tobacco and anti-alcohol messages among their peers.
   - Engage youth in the creation of media campaigns, ensuring messages resonate with their age group.
8. **Cultural Sensitivity Training:**
   - Provide cultural sensitivity training for law enforcement and regulators to ensure that efforts to combat underage sales do not inadvertently result in racial profiling or discriminatory practices.

9. **Data Collection and Research:**
   - Regularly gather data on sales patterns, youth smoking, and drinking rates in neighborhoods to assess the impact of interventions.
   - Fund research to understand the cultural, socioeconomic, and psychological factors that influence Urban youth's choices related to tobacco and alcohol.

10. **Collaboration:**
   - Foster collaborations between local governments, schools, nonprofits, parent groups, and business associations to form a united front against the underage sale and consumption of tobacco and alcohol.

By implementing these recommendations, communities can work towards safeguarding the health and well-being of their youth, ensuring they're protected from the premature influence of tobacco and alcohol.

Conclusion

Given the above findings, it's evident that neighborhood bodegas play a significant role in Urban youth's access to cigarettes and alcohol. The accessibility of cigarettes and alcohol to Urban youth via neighborhood bodegas is a multifaceted concern:

- Marketing Influence: Research underscores that adolescents' exposure to tobacco and alcohol marketing can influence their consumption behaviors. Receptivity to alcohol marketing predicts the initiation of alcohol use among adolescents. Similarly, the visibility of cigarette marketing within stores frequented by adolescents is prevalent. Such aggressive in-store marketing strategies can render neighborhood bodegas as powerful conduits through which youth, particularly Urban youth, are introduced to and enticed by these harmful products.

- Proximity to Educational Institutions: The density and location of tobacco retailers can further exacerbate this issue. There's a concerning link between the density of tobacco retailers near schools and increased tobacco use among students. This proximity allows for easier access, especially during breaks or after school hours, and can normalize the purchase of these products among peer groups.

- Sales Practices and Law Enforcement: The enforcement, or lack thereof, of age-restriction laws in these bodegas poses an additional challenge. An increase in tobacco outlet density is associated with higher retailer cigarette sales without proper ID checks. This lax enforcement of underage tobacco laws, combined with the implicit validation from in-store marketing, can shape youths' beliefs and attitudes toward smoking. Moreover, the importance of considering various measures when evaluating adolescents' exposure to cigarette marketing in stores suggests that understanding this exposure can be instrumental in formulating policies to curb underage sales.

The accessibility of cigarettes and alcohol to Urban youth via neighborhood bodegas is indeed a multifaceted concern. Addressing this issue necessitates a comprehensive understanding of these dynamics, including the marketing, density, and sales practices of bodegas, and requires concerted efforts from both policymakers and community stakeholders to mitigate the associated risks.

Chapter 7: Bodegas and Urban Youth Health: Seeking Positive Change

Introduction

Bodegas are integral to the fabric of many urban neighborhoods, offering residents convenience and familiarity. However, these establishments have come under scrutiny for their role in promoting unhealthy eating habits among urban youth, primarily due to a preponderance of processed foods and sugary beverages and a dearth of healthier alternatives.

The Impact on Urban Youth's Health

The dietary choices available in urban settings, especially those presented in bodegas, play a pivotal role in shaping the health trajectories of the residents, most notably the youth. The prominence of bodegas in many urban landscapes means that they become crucial access points for daily sustenance. Borradaile et al. (2009) have illuminated how snack food displays in such corner stores can trigger impulse purchases, often leading to choices that are high in calories, sugar, and sodium. The over-reliance on such nutrient-poor choices sets the stage for significant dietary imbalances.

Recommended Community-Based Interventions

Community organizations have the potential to lead proactive initiatives addressing dietary disparities in urban settings. Through the orchestration of health promotion events like community health fairs, they can spread essential knowledge about nutrition (Gottlieb & Joshi, 2010). Partnering with local educational institutions can also ensure that nutrition education becomes an integral part of the school curriculum, thus reaching the younger demographic in a more structured manner (Ravitch, 2010).

Recognizing the significant role that bodegas play in the dietary habits of urban communities, fostering partnerships with these establishments can make a transformative difference. Collaborative endeavors with bodega owners can pave the way for the inclusion of healthier food items in their stock (Borradaile et al., 2009). A possible incentive to encourage this transition might involve providing tax reductions or subsidies to bodegas that maintain a specific quota of healthy food offerings (Laska et al., 2010).

Fresh produce initiatives can also have a lasting impact. The establishment of community gardens not only empowers residents to grow their fresh produce but also provides bodegas with an accessible source of fresh foods (Reynolds & Cohen, 2016). These efforts can be complemented by hosting regular farmers' markets, which can both offer residents diverse food choices and motivate bodegas to invest in local and healthier food sources (Walker, Keane, & Burke, 2010).

A "Healthy Bodega" certification program could further steer bodegas towards healthier practices. By meeting certain health-focused criteria, bodegas can earn this certification, making them more attractive to a growing number of health-aware customers and potentially increasing their profitability (Powell et al., 2007).

It's imperative to remember the influential role of the youth in shaping the community's dietary patterns. Incorporating them in the decision-making processes can ensure that their unique needs and perspectives are considered (Henriksen et al., 2004). Community-led initiatives can support youth-driven campaigns that shed light on the significance of a balanced diet and underscore the health consequences of over-relying on processed foods (Kumanyika, 2008).

Church-Led Interventions

Churches, by virtue of their role as community anchors, are uniquely positioned to advocate for healthier dietary practices within their congregations and wider communities. By hosting nutritional workshops, they provide an essential platform for members, including the youth, to grasp the intricacies of balanced diets, understand the nuances of food labels, and discern how to make healthier choices in local bodegas (Kumanyika, 2008). Recognizing the crucial role bodegas serve in providing urban communities with their daily nourishment (Borradaile et al., 2009; Laska et al., 2010), churches can engage proactively with bodega owners. Through collective buying power, they could purchase healthier products in bulk, thereby negotiating lower prices and enhancing the accessibility of nutritious foods for the community (Larson et al., 2009).

Leveraging the vast spaces many churches possess, the establishment of community gardens becomes feasible (Reynolds & Cohen, 2016; White, 2011). Not only does this practice offer a direct source of fresh produce for community members, but it can also serve as a potential supply chain for bodegas, fostering a symbiotic relationship (Walker, Keane, & Burke, 2010).

By organizing health fairs, churches can double down on their commitment to holistic well-being. Such platforms are not just educational – offering insights into the implications of dietary choices (Gottlieb & Joshi, 2010) – but can also become sites where professionals, like nutritionists and doctors, render their expertise, offering the community valuable advice and health screenings (Powell et al., 2007).

Strengthening community ties, churches can facilitate events focused on the exchange of healthy recipes. These gatherings, while promoting nutritious and affordable meals that can be prepared using items commonly available in bodegas (Laska et al., 2010), also become a testament to community spirit, fostering stronger bonds and camaraderie among members.

Engagement of the youth remains one of the most potent avenues through which churches can amplify their health advocacy efforts (Henriksen et al., 2004). Enlisting them in activities ranging from gardening to health fair organization, churches not only equip them with essential life skills and

knowledge but also position them as influential advocates.
These young individuals, with their energy and connectivity,
can resonate with their peers, driving home the importance of
healthy dietary practices and becoming beacons of change
within their communities (Grier & Kumanyika, 2008).

Potential Challenges

Bodega owners, who play a crucial role in the food
environments of urban communities, may harbor reservations
about altering their product offerings, fearing reduced profits
from potentially slower-selling healthier items (Borradaile et
al., 2009; Larson et al., 2009). Such concerns may stem from a
lack of awareness about the adverse health implications of
some products commonly found in these stores, coupled with
the perception that introducing healthier products may not be
economically viable (Grier & Kumanyika, 2008; Cummins &
Macintyre, 2006).

The shift towards a healthier product lineup could be
seen as financially risky, particularly given the entrenched
purchasing habits of longtime customers (Walker, Keane, &
Burke, 2010). Yet, interventions like subsidies or incentives
could alleviate some of these financial concerns, making it
more appealing for bodega owners to consider stocking
healthier options (Laska et al., 2010; Powell et al., 2007).

Additionally, while initial resistance from some
consumers might be expected, persistent community
engagement and education can potentially reshape purchasing
behaviors over time. Raising awareness about the health
consequences of certain products and championing the

benefits of healthier alternatives can play a pivotal role in shifting community preferences (Kumanyika, 2008; Morland et al., 2002).

Conclusion

Community institutions, including churches and local organizations, have an instrumental role in shaping the health trajectories of urban youth. By forging partnerships with bodegas, which serve as integral community fixtures, these entities can collaboratively work towards enhancing the health landscape of urban settings. Despite the intrinsic value of bodegas to urban communities, there's a growing awareness of their potential negative impact on the health of young city dwellers, particularly due to the availability of impulse snack foods and other unhealthy products.

Religious institutions, like churches, which have historically played transformative roles in urban communities, are uniquely positioned to galvanize efforts that promote healthier dietary choices. With their influential status, churches can encourage bodegas to transition from being perceived as health liabilities to becoming esteemed collaborators committed to bolstering community health and vitality.

Chapter 8: Guarding Kids from Bodega Health Risks: A Parent's Guide

Introduction

Bodegas, or corner stores, are ubiquitous in many urban areas and provide a convenient option for shopping, especially for families without immediate access to larger grocery stores. While they offer convenience, many bodegas stock a high proportion of processed foods, sugary beverages, and other unhealthy options. As a result, frequent reliance on bodegas can contribute to poor dietary habits among children. This chapter highlights strategies that parents can employ to mitigate the negative health impacts associated with frequenting bodegas.

Understanding the Issue

Bodegas, especially those located in urban areas, tend to prioritize stocking items that boast extended shelf lives, such as processed foods (Borradaile et al., 2009; Larson, Story, & Nelson, 2009). One of the challenges these stores face is the perishability of fresh produce compared to the longevity of processed items (Laska et al., 2010). Consequently, the products available in these stores frequently contain high amounts of sugar, salt, and unhealthy fats (Gottlieb & Joshi, 2010). The implications of such dietary patterns are concerning, with evidence suggesting that consistent consumption of these processed foods can elevate the risk of health complications, including obesity (Kumanyika, 2008), diabetes (Cummins & Macintyre, 2006), and cardiovascular diseases (Morland et al., 2002).

Strategies for Parents

1. **Educate and Communicate:** The foundation of instilling healthy habits in children starts with clear communication. Initiate discussions with your children about what constitutes a balanced diet, including the benefits of consuming whole, nutrient-rich foods and the drawbacks of overly processed ones.

   Use age-appropriate examples and analogies to explain the body's need for different nutrients, akin to how a car requires the right fuel to run efficiently. Highlight the dangers of excessive sugar, preservatives, and unhealthy fats found in many products at bodegas. Share relatable stories or documentaries that shed light on the long-term health consequences of an imbalanced diet, such as obesity, diabetes, and heart diseases.

   Furthermore, engage in interactive activities, like reading food labels together during shopping trips, to reinforce these lessons and promote informed food choices.

Remember, it's not about instilling fear but empowering them with knowledge to make better decisions.

2. **Plan Ahead:** One of the best strategies to ensure your family maintains a balanced diet is proactive planning. Instead of relying solely on the convenience of nearby bodegas, set aside time for visits to larger supermarkets or farmers' markets where a diverse range of fresh produce, lean meats, whole grains, and other nutritious options are available. Before each trip, take a moment to assess what your household needs for the upcoming days or week.

    Involve your children in the process of creating a shopping list, allowing them to suggest meals or snacks they'd like. This not only keeps them engaged but also serves as an educational opportunity to discuss the nutritional value of their choices. By sticking to a well-thought-out list, you reduce the likelihood of diverting to unhealthy impulse buys, especially when children are enticed by colorful packaging or promotional offers.

    Additionally, having a list aids in budgeting and ensures you have all the ingredients necessary for healthier home-cooked meals, minimizing the need for last-minute runs to the bodega.

3. **Cook Together:** Engaging children in the culinary process can be a transformative experience for their relationship with food. By inviting them into the kitchen, you're granting them an opportunity to witness firsthand the journey of ingredients from raw materials to the final dish on their plate. Through this involvement, they gain a deeper appreciation for the various foods and how they contribute to a wholesome meal.

Teaching them about each ingredient—where it comes from, its nutritional benefits, and its role in the dish—provides them with valuable knowledge they can carry into adulthood. Furthermore, children often exhibit a sense of pride and accomplishment when they've had a hand in crafting a meal. This emotional connection can make them more enthusiastic about consuming dishes that are both tasty and nutritious.

Additionally, cooking together fosters family bonding, promotes experimentation with diverse recipes and cuisines, and instills essential life skills. Over time, as they gain confidence and knowledge, children will be better equipped to make healthier food choices, even when faced with the tempting array of less nutritious options at local bodegas.

4. **Limit Bodega Visits:** Bodegas, with their convenient locations and array of products, often become a regular stop for many urban families. However, given the potential health risks associated with the frequent consumption of processed foods and sugary beverages commonly found in these stores, it's prudent to manage how often you and your children visit.

By planning your shopping trips in advance and stocking up on essentials from larger grocery stores, you can reduce the reliance on bodegas for daily needs. When circumstances require a bodega visit, take it as an opportunity to educate your children. Walk through the aisles together, comparing products, reading labels, and discussing the nutritional value of different items. This hands-on approach helps children discern between healthier choices and less nutritious temptations.

Over time, with consistent guidance, they'll develop the habit of gravitating towards the healthiest options available, even in environments where those choices might be limited. Such skills not only protect them from the immediate health concerns associated with poor diet but also set the foundation for a lifetime of informed eating habits.

5. **Advocate for Healthier Options:** Building a rapport with local bodega owners can be a proactive step towards introducing healthier food alternatives in these establishments. As a regular customer, your opinions and preferences hold value. Initiate conversations with store owners about the health benefits of stocking more nutritious products, sharing insights about the growing consumer demand for such options.

   Highlight that there's a community of parents and concerned individuals who are seeking healthier choices for their children, and that there's potential for increased business from catering to this demand. Additionally, pooling requests with other like-minded parents or community members can make your collective voice stronger, emphasizing the broader desire for change. Remember, bodega owners operate businesses, and they respond to market demands.

   By consistently advocating for more wholesome products and supporting these products with your purchases, you not only safeguard the health of your children but also contribute to a positive shift in community eating habits. Over time, as more customers echo similar sentiments, bodegas may progressively modify their inventory to

reflect the community's evolving preferences, leading to a
win-win situation for both store owners and consumers.

6. **Lead by Example:** One of the most influential teaching
    tools a parent possesses is their own behavior. Children,
    especially at younger ages, tend to mirror the habits and
    choices of those they look up to, primarily their parents.
    When you consistently prioritize healthy eating choices, it
    sends a powerful message to your children about the
    importance of nutrition and well-being.

    Whether you're at a bodega, a supermarket, or dining out,
    consciously opt for nutritious meals and snacks. For
    instance, instead of reaching for a soda at the bodega,
    choose water or a natural juice. Opt for whole grain
    products over heavily processed ones, and pick fresh
    fruits as snacks instead of sugary confections. When
    children observe these choices regularly, they internalize
    the value of such decisions.

    Additionally, openly discuss your reasoning behind these
    choices with your children, allowing them to understand
    the "why" behind the action. This not only establishes a
    pattern of healthy eating but also fosters an environment
    of informed decision-making. Over time, these consistent
    demonstrations act as silent lessons, shaping your
    children's perceptions and preferences towards food,
    making them more inclined to naturally gravitate towards
    healthier options as they grow.

7. **Encourage Hydration with Water:** One of the
    significant pitfalls in many modern diets, especially among
    children, is the heavy consumption of sugary beverages
    like sodas, energy drinks, and even some misleading

"fruit" juices. These drinks often contribute to a high intake of empty calories, which means they add to the calorie count without providing any real nutritional value. Over time, regular consumption of such beverages can lead to weight gain, dental problems, and increased risks of chronic diseases.

Educating children about these risks is essential, but so is presenting the positive benefits of drinking water. Water plays a critical role in almost every function within our bodies. From regulating body temperature to aiding digestion and flushing out toxins, water is a vital component of maintaining good health. By teaching children about the myriad functions and benefits of water, they can begin to appreciate its importance.

Moreover, it's essential to make water more appealing. Parents can invest in fun, reusable water bottles, or even flavor water with slices of natural fruits like cucumber, lemon, or strawberries for a hint of taste without added sugars. Making a habit of always having a bottle of water on hand, especially when out and about, can help reinforce its importance.

Additionally, families can set hydration goals or challenges to motivate children to drink more water. For example, setting a goal to drink eight glasses of water a day and tracking progress together can make the process more interactive and fun. Through consistent encouragement and by showcasing the tangible benefits, parents can instill a preference for water over sugary alternatives in their children, setting them on a path to healthier hydration habits.

8. **Seek Alternatives:** In today's fast-paced world, the allure
   of quick, accessible snacks like chips or candies is
   undeniable, especially for children. These snacks, often
   high in salt, sugar, and unhealthy fats, can quickly become
   a dietary staple if not checked. However, by introducing
   and promoting healthier alternatives, parents can ensure
   that their children develop better eating habits from a
   young age.

   Fruits, for instance, are nature's candies. They come
   packed with essential vitamins, minerals, and fiber, all of
   which are crucial for a child's growth and development.
   Nuts, on the other hand, are rich in proteins, healthy fats,
   and antioxidants. By encouraging children to snack on a
   handful of almonds, walnuts, or even roasted chickpeas,
   parents can provide them with sustained energy and vital
   nutrients without the excessive sugars and salts.

   To make this transition smoother, it's important to have a
   consistent stock of these healthier alternatives at home.
   This means setting aside a designated snack drawer or
   shelf filled with an assortment of dried fruits, mixed nuts,
   yogurt, and perhaps even dark chocolate for those
   occasional cravings. Pre-packaged portions of these
   snacks can be prepared for on-the-go situations, ensuring
   children always have a healthy option within arm's reach.

   Furthermore, making these snacks appealing is key. This
   can be achieved through creative presentation. For
   example, fruit kabobs, nut butter dips, or yogurt parfaits
   can make snacking both fun and nutritious. Parents can
   also involve their children in the preparation process,
   letting them choose their mix of fruits or nuts, thereby
   giving them a sense of autonomy over their food choices.

Lastly, it's essential to communicate the benefits of these healthier alternatives. By understanding why these snacks are better for their health, children are more likely to make better food decisions independently. Over time, as they develop a palate for these wholesome foods, the allure of processed snacks will diminish, leading to a lifetime of healthier eating habits.

9. **Community Engagement:** In the effort to instill healthy eating habits among children, there's strength in numbers. By uniting with other parents and community members, a collective force can be harnessed to create a larger, more influential impact on children's dietary choices. Engaging at the community level offers a multifaceted approach to reinforcing the importance of nutrition and ensuring children grow up with a balanced understanding of food and its implications on their health.

Firstly, community collaboration can lead to the organization of events or workshops tailored to the local demographic. For example, a neighborhood could host a "Healthy Food Fair," where local chefs or nutritionists demonstrate easy-to-make, nutritious recipes. Kids can participate in hands-on cooking sessions, turning education into a fun, interactive experience. This approach not only teaches children about nutrition but also equips them with basic culinary skills they can use throughout their lives.

Additionally, group discussions or workshops can be organized where parents can share tips, strategies, and recipes that have worked for their families. These sessions could also include expert talks from nutritionists, dietitians, or pediatricians, providing parents with the knowledge and resources to make informed decisions about their children's diet.

Engaging with schools is another effective strategy. Parents can collaborate to introduce or strengthen school programs focused on nutrition education. By partnering with teachers and school administrators, parents can ensure that the message of healthy eating is consistently reinforced both at home and in school.

Moreover, community engagement can extend beyond educational events. Parents can come together to create community gardens, providing a local source of fresh, organic produce. These gardens can serve as hands-on learning centers for children, teaching them about agriculture, sustainability, and the benefits of consuming fresh, unprocessed foods.

Finally, community-driven petitions or campaigns can be initiated to encourage local bodegas or stores to stock healthier food options. A collective voice, representing a significant portion of their customer base, will likely prompt store owners to reconsider their inventory, catering more to the health-conscious demands of the community.

In summary, when parents and community members join forces, their combined efforts can lead to a profound shift in the community's health culture. Such engagement not only promotes healthy eating habits among children but also fosters a sense of unity and shared responsibility towards the well-being of the younger generation.

Conclusion

Bodegas, deeply rooted in many urban landscapes, serve as more than just convenience stores; they become essential to community life, often turning into local landmarks and gathering places. However, despite their critical community role, these establishments often stock a multitude of processed and sugary food options, which can significantly influence the dietary preferences of the youth.

The responsibility of molding a child's eating habits primarily lies with the parents, especially during the formative early years when lasting dietary habits take root. While offerings from places like bodegas certainly influence choices, the family environment and guidance from parents are paramount.

To truly guide their children, parents must be proactive, not just reactive. This could involve preparing nutritious snacks to counter the allure of less healthy alternatives or continuously highlighting the benefits of wholesome foods over processed options. Creating an environment where making healthier choices feels natural and appealing is essential.

Children often mirror the behaviors they see, especially from influential figures like their parents. Watching a parent choose a healthy apple over chips or water over soda can be more educational than any lecture.

Furthermore, imparting dietary wisdom isn't just about setting rules. It involves open conversations where children's thoughts are valued, their desires recognized, and the societal pressures they face are understood. By empathetically presenting healthier options, parents can ensure their children feel heard and understood, rather than restricted. Here, nutritional guidance becomes a two-way conversation, enriching mutual understanding.

In summary, while bodegas and other external factors undeniably influence dietary choices, the role parents play is incomparable. By actively demonstrating positive dietary practices and creating an open, educational atmosphere, parents can guide their children towards healthier lives. Through this effort, they not only benefit their immediate family but also set the groundwork for healthier future generations, resilient against the ebb and flow of dietary temptations.

Chapter 9: Urban Children's Preference: Bodega vs. Cafeteria Food

Introduction

Bodegas, small convenience stores typically found in urban areas, are a primary source of food for many urban children. Despite efforts by schools to provide nutritious meals in cafeterias, numerous children prefer to get their meals or snacks from these bodegas. This chapter explores the reasons behind this preference.

Cultural Relevance and Variety

Bodegas, intrinsic components of urban landscapes, typically provide a diverse range of food products tailored to cater to the palates of the local population. Notably, the offerings at these establishments often encompass ethnic and cultural foods, which stand as reflections of the community's heritage and culinary inclinations (Morland et al., 2002; Walker, Keane, & Burke, 2010). Such diversity can be crucial, especially in neighborhoods marked by racial and cultural richness, where access to culturally relevant foods can be a significant determinant of food choices (Williams, 2006).

In stark contrast, school cafeterias often operate within the constraints of set menus, primarily driven by budgetary considerations, federal guidelines, and the challenges of mass food production (Ravitch, 2010). These menus, though designed to be nutritionally balanced, might lack the breadth of ethnic and cultural representation. As a result, they may not be reflective of students' home cuisines or the dietary preferences shaped by their cultural backgrounds (Kumanyika, 2008). This limited cultural diversity in cafeteria offerings could inadvertently sideline the diverse culinary traditions present within the student population, thus making the allure of bodegas even stronger.

Furthermore, the broader urban food environment plays a pivotal role in shaping dietary behaviors. While some areas may be food deserts, lacking in access to healthy food options (Larson, Story, & Nelson, 2009; Powell et al., 2007), Bodegas often fill these gaps, serving as vital food access points in such neighborhoods (Laska et al., 2010). However, the implications of such accessibility can be multifaceted. On one hand, Bodegas offer culturally relevant food choices; on the other, they might also display a plethora of snack foods which can trigger impulse purchases, potentially contributing to unhealthy dietary patterns among urban children (Borradaile et al., 2009).

In conclusion, the interplay between the offerings at bodegas and school cafeterias, set against the backdrop of a multifarious urban food environment, underscores the intricate nature of food choices made by urban children. Incorporating cultural and ethnic diversity in school cafeteria menus might not only make them more appealing but also serve as a step towards acknowledging and celebrating the diverse culinary traditions of the student community.

Convenience and Accessibility

Bodegas, a hallmark of urban landscapes, often serve as neighborhood hubs due to their strategic locations close to residential areas and schools (Morland et al., 2002; Laska et al., 2010). Their proximity to educational institutions makes them easily accessible to students both before and after the school hours (Borradaile et al., 2009). This strategic location, especially in areas facing disparities in access to healthy foods, ensures that bodegas play an essential role in food choices of the younger demographic (Larson, Story, & Nelson, 2009; Walker, Keane, & Burke, 2010).

The convenience offered by bodegas goes beyond their mere presence. Their small size and focused product range enable a quick in-and-out shopping experience. Contrastingly, school cafeterias, which are structured to serve a large number of students within a short time frame, often have long lines and considerable wait times, especially during peak lunch hours (Ravitch, 2010). This difference in service speed can make bodegas an attractive option for students looking for a quick snack or meal, especially given the hustle and bustle of urban life (Dubois, 1935).

Furthermore, the neighborhoods where bodegas are situated often reflect a diverse set of socio-economic and cultural backgrounds, with the products on their shelves mirroring these variances (Powell et al., 2007; White, 2011). This stands in stark contrast to the standardization seen in school cafeterias, which, while striving for nutritional balance, might not offer the same range of cultural or preference-based choices (Kumanyika, 2008).

The marketing strategies employed by bodegas also play a role in their appeal. Studies have shown that marketing is more prevalent in stores where adolescents shop frequently, with a range of products - from snacks to cigarettes - being strategically placed to attract youth (Henriksen et al., 2004; Feighery et al., 2006). The presence of such marketing techniques, combined with the implications of targeted food and beverage marketing to specific racial or ethnic groups, can also influence the choices made by urban children (Grier & Kumanyika, 2008).

In essence, the allure of bodegas for students revolves around convenience, proximity, product diversity, and marketing, all of which collectively offer a contrasting experience to the structured, time-consuming environment of school cafeterias.

Perception of Taste and Quality

For many students in urban settings, school cafeterias have garnered a reputation for serving meals that some perceive as bland or of inferior quality (Ravitch, 2010). This perception, whether accurate or not, can influence their food choices and drive them to alternative sources of sustenance. Bodegas, often found in close proximity to schools, emerge as convenient alternatives (Morland et al., 2002). While these establishments are known for their quick, in-and-out nature, the items they offer, especially those readily visible, are often aligned with impulse-purchase behaviors (Borradaile et al., 2009).

It's not just about the convenience; it's also about the appeal. Bodegas offer a myriad of flavorful and culturally diverse food options, resonating with the palates and preferences of urban youth (Laska et al., 2010; White, 2011). These foods, though often high in sugar, salt, and unhealthy fats, present an allure with their rich tastes and textures, making them seemingly more desirable than the perceived bland offerings of school cafeterias (Cummins & Macintyre, 2006).

Moreover, the targeted marketing strategies within these stores further amplify this appeal. Companies meticulously place snack foods and beverages to capture the attention of youth, capitalizing on their vulnerabilities and preferences (Grier & Kumanyika, 2008; Henriksen et al., 2004). Such tactics can overshadow the health implications of consuming these products, as the immediate sensory satisfaction often takes precedence for many young consumers (Gottlieb & Joshi, 2010).

The cultural context is also pivotal. In ethnically diverse urban settings, bodegas often cater to the specific tastes and preferences of their local communities, offering food items that resonate with cultural or familial traditions (Dubois, 1935; Kumanyika, 2008). For many students, this can be a comforting reminder of home, making the allure of bodegas even stronger.

However, it is essential to recognize that the food landscape's appeal isn't solely about taste or immediate satisfaction. It's deeply interwoven with socio-economic factors, racial dynamics, and historical implications (Coates, 2014; Williams, 2006). Areas with limited access to fresh and healthy foods, often termed "food deserts," can inadvertently push residents, including students, towards more readily available but less nutritious options (Walker, Keane, & Burke, 2010).

In summary, while school cafeterias strive to provide balanced meals, the combination of students' perceptions, bodega convenience, targeted marketing, cultural resonance, and broader socio-economic factors makes the choice of bodega foods compelling, if not always healthier.

Autonomy and Independence

Purchasing food from bodegas provides urban students a distinctive sense of autonomy and empowerment (Dubois, 1935). In the diverse landscape of urban America, bodegas stand as cornerstones of communities, offering an array of foods that often reflect the cultural preferences of the neighborhoods they serve (White, 2011; Gottlieb & Joshi, 2010). Within these establishments, students can exercise independence and decision-making by selecting foods that resonate with their cultural backgrounds or individual tastes (Kumanyika, 2008). This freedom to choose is not just about satiating hunger—it becomes an act of self-expression and agency.

Contrarily, school cafeterias, while essential in providing nutrition to students, often come with limitations. The array of choices can be constrained, influenced by budgetary considerations, nutritional guidelines, and mass-procurement strategies (Ravitch, 2010). Furthermore, the general perception among some students that cafeteria food is unappealing, bland, or of lower quality exacerbates this feeling of restriction (Larson, Story, & Nelson, 2009).

Bodegas, however, might not always be the healthier alternative. Their shelves often prioritize snack foods and products that trigger impulse purchases, further enticing young buyers (Borradaile et al., 2009). The appeal of these foods is magnified by targeted marketing strategies, which are meticulously designed to capture the attention of the youth, making them more prone to making less-than-optimal dietary choices (Grier & Kumanyika, 2008; Henriksen et al., 2004).

Yet, it is the very act of choosing, of asserting one's preferences, that makes bodegas alluring to students. In the broader socio-economic and racial contexts, the act of choosing food, even from a bodega, can be seen as a form of resistance or empowerment, especially in neighborhoods marked by food deserts or areas with limited access to fresh and healthy foods (Coates, 2014; Walker, Keane, & Burke, 2010). For many students, walking into a bodega and selecting a snack or a drink becomes a small yet significant act of agency, in contrast to the perceived constraints of the school food environment (Williams, 2006).

In summary, while school cafeterias play a vital role in student nutrition, the allure of bodegas lies not just in the range of products they offer but in the autonomy they provide to students. The freedom to choose, even in the simple act of selecting a snack, reflects deeper socio-cultural dynamics and the inherent human desire for agency and self-expression.

Peer Influence

Bodega visits serve as more than just a pitstop for urban youth; they often represent a nexus of social interaction and cultural expression (Dubois, 1935). The act of visiting bodegas can be deeply rooted in the urban tapestry, offering students a place not only to buy food but also to hang out and engage in social activities with peers (Gottlieb & Joshi, 2010). With bodegas commonly located in close proximity to urban schools and residential areas, they easily become regular meeting spots for students after school hours (Morland et al., 2002; Larson, Story, & Nelson, 2009).

The allure of bodegas isn't limited to the availability of diverse food options alone. Their role as communal spaces can lead to significant peer influence. With the bodega culture so intertwined with urban youth's daily life, there's an inherent pressure to fit into the social fabric by partaking in popular food choices, even if these choices are not the healthiest (Borradaile et al., 2009). Peer pressure and the desire for social acceptance can amplify consumption patterns. For instance, if a popular snack is trending among friends, a student might feel an intrinsic need to try it too, regardless of its nutritional value, in a bid to fit in (Kumanyika, 2008).

While school cafeterias might strive to offer a balance of nutritional options, they often lack the allure of novel and culturally diverse products available at bodegas (Laska et al., 2010). Moreover, the marketing strategies employed by bodegas, intentionally or otherwise, target this younger audience, making them more susceptible to impulse purchases, especially when accompanied by peers (Grier & Kumanyika, 2008; Henriksen et al., 2004).

However, it's essential to note that while bodegas offer an essential cultural and social space for urban students, they might also inadvertently expose students to other risk factors. With the higher prevalence of cigarette and alcohol marketing in stores frequently visited by adolescents, there's a risk of normalization of such products in their perceptions (Feighery et al., 2006; Henriksen et al., 2008).

In summary, the bodega's significance in the urban landscape goes beyond just food offerings. It represents a microcosm of urban youth culture, interwoven with elements of peer interaction, cultural expression, and social dynamics (White, 2011; Coates, 2014). While these spaces offer students a sense of community and identity, they also bring forth challenges related to dietary choices and potential exposure to other risk factors.

Limited Awareness of Nutrition

Bodegas, corner stores typically found in urban areas, often act as vital food sources for many residents, including students (Borradaile et al., 2009). The ubiquity of bodegas, coupled with their convenience, makes them popular spots for young people looking for quick and accessible food options. However, this accessibility comes at a cost, particularly concerning the quality and nutritional value of available food items.

Many of the products stocked by bodegas are high in sugar, fat, and salt (Borradaile et al., 2009). This high-calorie, low-nutrient food environment can have serious implications for the health of consumers, particularly young students. Cummins & Macintyre (2006) suggest that such food environments contribute significantly to the prevalence of obesity, not only at the neighborhood level but also on a national scale. This phenomenon is exacerbated by the fact that healthier food options are often less accessible in urban areas, contributing to what many refer to as "food deserts" (Walker, R. E., Keane, C. R., & Burke, J. G., 2010).

There are significant disparities in access to healthy foods in the U.S., with socio-economic factors and race playing crucial roles (Larson, Story, & Nelson, 2009; Williams, 2006). The strategic positioning of unhealthy food items and the scarcity of nutritious alternatives in bodegas can be linked to targeted food and beverage marketing towards specific demographic groups, particularly African Americans (Grier & Kumanyika, 2008). Such targeting practices, combined with socio-economic pressures, can further alienate marginalized communities from healthy food access.

Students, in particular, might not always be fully aware of the nutritional implications of their food choices (Gottlieb & Joshi, 2010). With the bombardment of advertising and the appeal of tasty, high-sugar, and high-fat snacks, many may choose these over healthier cafeteria options, even if they are available. Furthermore, peer influence and the allure of popular, culturally resonant snacks can further skew their choices towards these less nutritious options (Kumanyika, 2008). This is not to mention the broader societal implications of food justice and how socio-economic dynamics dictate access to healthy food (Reynolds & Cohen, 2016).

The role of bodegas in urban food landscapes is complex. On one hand, they offer convenience and cultural touchpoints for many city dwellers. On the other hand, they often perpetuate unhealthy food consumption patterns, especially among young students. To shift these patterns, a deeper understanding of urban food systems, their historical contexts, and the socio-economic forces at play is necessary (Dubois, 1935; Coates, 2014; White, 2011).

Pricing and Affordability

Bodegas, small convenience stores often found in urban neighborhoods, have evolved into significant fixtures of the urban food landscape, especially for the youth. Their accessibility and the range of products they offer often make them a preferred choice for many, including students (Borradaile et al., 2009).

One notable aspect of bodegas is their pricing strategies. To appeal to a broad customer base, especially those with limited purchasing power, bodegas often offer competitive prices, deals, or bulk purchasing options on specific items (Laska et al., 2010). For students, particularly those with constrained budgets, these pricing dynamics can make bodegas more attractive than school cafeterias. Even though school meals can be subsidized or entirely free, the perception of getting more value for money at a bodega can outweigh the benefits of a potentially healthier school meal (Larson, Story, & Nelson, 2009).

The neighborhood food environments further exacerbate this scenario. Many urban neighborhoods face significant disparities in access to healthy foods, creating "food deserts" where residents, especially those from marginalized communities, have limited choices (Walker, Keane, & Burke, 2010). In such environments, bodegas might be one of the few accessible sources of food, even if the options they offer are not always the healthiest (Morland et al., 2002; Powell et al., 2007). The consequence of this is that while school meals might be designed to offer balanced nutrition, the allure of perceived better deals and more varied options in bodegas can often overshadow these meals (Gottlieb & Joshi, 2010).

Furthermore, the influence of targeted marketing can't be overlooked. Companies often target their products, especially high-sugar, high-fat snacks, to specific demographics, particularly to young people and ethnic minorities (Grier & Kumanyika, 2008; Kumanyika, 2008). These targeted efforts can make certain products more appealing, further driving students to opt for bodegas over school meals. This dynamic is not limited to food alone. For instance, Henriksen and colleagues (2004; 2008) have shown how marketing strategies for cigarettes and alcohol are more prevalent in stores frequented by adolescents, demonstrating the power of targeted marketing.

Bodegas also exist within broader urban, socio-economic, and racial contexts. The challenges faced by urban neighborhoods, from poverty to systemic racism, have repercussions on how residents, including students, interact with their food environments (Williams, 2006; Dubois, 1935). The appeal of bodegas, with their competitive prices and deals, might not merely be a matter of personal preference but a reflection of larger systemic challenges that many urban residents face.

In conclusion, while bodegas offer convenience and often economically appealing choices, understanding their popularity among students requires a nuanced consideration of urban food landscapes, marketing strategies, and socio-economic factors. Schools and policymakers need to understand and address these dynamics to ensure that students are making the healthiest choices for their well-being (Coates, 2014; Ravitch, 2010).

Packaging and Marketing

Bodegas and small urban convenience stores have become pivotal points of food acquisition in urban environments, especially for younger individuals. One of the primary appeals of bodegas is the variety of commercial snacks they offer, which often sport vibrant, eye-catching packaging. Borradaile et al. (2009) highlighted the pervasive availability of snack food displays in corner stores in Philadelphia that can potentially trigger impulse purchases. Such displays, combined with the aggressive marketing campaigns behind these products, are specifically tailored to captivate the attention of younger consumers (Grier & Kumanyika, 2008).

The allure of these snacks goes beyond just the packaging. The products themselves are frequently tied to expansive advertising campaigns that saturate television, the internet, and other media platforms that young people engage with (Kumanyika, 2008). The magnitude of this exposure means that when adolescents or young adults walk into a bodega, they're not just seeing a snack; they're seeing a product they've been conditioned to recognize and desire due to repeated exposure to its advertisement.

Contrastingly, the food available in school cafeterias often comes in plain packaging, and the meal options might not always be as immediately gratifying to the palate as some commercial snacks. The lack of targeted marketing and branding for cafeteria foods further dims their allure, making them seem less enticing when compared to the brightly packaged, heavily advertised snacks in bodegas (Larson, Story, & Nelson, 2009).

Moreover, it's not just the food industry that uses these aggressive marketing tactics in locations frequented by the youth. Similar strategies are employed in the tobacco and alcohol industries. For instance, Henriksen et al. (2004; 2008) found a significant presence of cigarette and alcohol marketing in stores where adolescents shopped frequently, demonstrating the broader tactic of targeting young consumers at the point of sale.

The broader food environment plays a significant role in shaping these preferences. Disparities in access to healthy foods often mean that bodegas become primary food sources for many urban residents (Walker, Keane, & Burke, 2010). This reliance on bodegas for food acquisition, combined with aggressive marketing strategies, makes commercial snacks even more prominent in the diets of urban youth. Additionally, factors like racial and socioeconomic dynamics can further influence food choices. Williams (2006) elaborated on the intersections of race, socioeconomic status, and health, suggesting that systemic factors, including targeted advertising, play a role in perpetuating health disparities in marginalized communities.

Furthermore, the historical and socio-cultural context of urban environments, as discussed by Dubois (1935) and Coates (2014), also intertwines with contemporary food dynamics, creating a complex web where food choices are influenced by a mix of marketing, availability, and deeper systemic issues.

In summary, the appeal of commercial snacks in bodegas goes beyond just eye-catching packaging. It's a confluence of aggressive marketing, disparities in food availability, and broader socio-cultural factors that make these products more attractive to young consumers than the seemingly mundane options available in school cafeterias. Addressing this issue requires a holistic understanding of urban food landscapes and the forces that shape them.

Recommendations

- **Improve Cafeteria Offerings:** Schools can diversify their menu to incorporate more culturally relevant foods and improve the taste and presentation of meals.

- **Nutritional Education:** Schools should invest in nutrition education to help students make healthier choices both inside and outside school.

- **Engage Students:** Schools can involve students in menu planning or introduce cooking clubs, which can pique interest in wholesome, home-cooked-style meals.

- **Bridge the Gap:** Collaborate with local bodegas to stock healthier options and provide students with discounts or incentives to choose those options.

Conclusion

Understanding urban children's preference for bodega food over cafeteria offerings provides insight into their food choices, revealing a complex interplay between marketing, environment, culture, and access.

One primary reason for the appeal of bodega snacks is their strategic presentation in stores. A prevalent display of snack foods in corner stores in Philadelphia is positioned to stimulate impulse purchases. These displays, paired with vibrant packaging, can easily draw a child's attention.

Beyond just the display, these commercial snacks are embedded within aggressive advertising campaigns that target younger consumers. Targeted food and beverage marketing can impact health outcomes, especially among African Americans. The repeated exposure to these marketing tactics can create a heightened attraction to such products when seen in stores.

In contrast, school cafeteria foods lack such marketing backing. They often come in plain packaging, and without promotional campaigns to glamorize them, they might seem less appealing than their commercial counterparts.

The wider food environment also plays a crucial role in this preference. Food environments can influence obesity trends. Often, urban areas have limited access to fresh and healthy food choices, with bodegas or small convenience stores becoming primary food sources. This limited access, compounded with aggressive marketing tactics, can amplify the appeal of bodega snacks.

Moreover, neighborhood characteristics influence the location and types of food stores available. If a neighborhood lacks full-service grocery stores but has an abundance of bodegas, children will naturally become more accustomed to the products these stores offer.

Furthermore, cultural and racial dynamics intersect with these preferences. The added health effects come with racism and discrimination. Urban areas, with their diverse populations, might find cultural food preferences merging with what's available, which in many urban environments is the bodega.

Interestingly, while bodegas present a challenge in terms of nutrition, they also represent a potential avenue for intervention. Healthy food availability in small urban food stores across US cities suggests that with the right strategies, these stores could be leveraged to promote better eating habits.

In conclusion, understanding urban children's food preferences is multifaceted, stemming from a combination of marketing, availability, cultural nuances, and broader socio-economic factors. Recognizing these dynamics allows schools and communities to make informed decisions to enhance the health and well-being of their students, whether through educational programs, cafeteria reforms, or community-based initiatives.

Chapter 10: Urban Parents' Case Against Bodegas for Unhealthy Child Targeting

Introduction

In the heart of urban environments, bodegas are a common sight, providing convenience and accessibility to various food products. However, there is increasing concern over the role they play in promoting unhealthy dietary habits among children. This chapter outlines the reasons why urban parents should consider a class action lawsuit against bodegas, as well as steps parents can follow to pursue legal action, for their alleged marketing practices targeting children with unhealthy foods.

Proliferation of Unhealthy Products

Bodegas often have an extensive array of unhealthy, processed foods high in sugar, salt, and unhealthy fats (Laska et al., 2010). Due to their addictive properties and taste, these products are particularly enticing for children (Kumanyika,

2008). These items are strategically marketed, with unhealthy snacks placed at eye level to catch a child's attention, encouraging impulse purchases (Borradaile et al., 2009). Additionally, these small-scale stores frequently offer promotions, particularly in the hours immediately after school, and some even partner with major brands to display products in appealing packaging or provide toy giveaways (Henriksen et al., 2004).

Constant consumption of these unhealthy products has significant health implications. Urban areas are experiencing increasing rates of childhood obesity, a trend driven in part by the easy access to these unhealthy choices (Larson, Story, & Nelson, 2009). Regular intake can lead to various health problems, including diabetes, dental issues, and cardiovascular diseases (Grier & Kumanyika, 2008).

While larger supermarket chains are often criticized for their role in promoting unhealthy foods, bodegas, due to their smaller size, escape similar scrutiny (Powell et al., 2007). Yet, considering their abundance and proximity to schools and residential areas, their influence is undeniable (Morland et al., 2002).

Children's dietary habits are greatly influenced by their immediate environment. For many urban youth, bodegas are the primary source of food, emphasizing the need for these establishments to be held accountable for promoting poor food choices (Walker, Keane, & Burke, 2010).

Economically, while bodegas might argue they are simply meeting demand, the societal costs of addressing health issues arising from poor diets can be significant (Gottlieb & Joshi, 2010). Over time, these societal costs may surpass the immediate profits made from selling these products (Williams, 2006).

Legal action could set a precedent, leading to:

- Regulations on the marketing and sale of unhealthy products for children (Feighery et al., 2006).
- Encouraging bodegas to stock healthier options (Laska et al., 2010).
- Campaigns promoting the importance of healthy eating (Gottlieb & Joshi, 2010).

In essence, children's health and well-being are paramount. Recognizing the influential role bodegas play in shaping children's diets underscores the importance of legal action as a means to promote healthier food environments in urban settings and protect future generations from preventable health issues.

Steps to Filing a Class Action Lawsuit Over Unhealthy Food Sales:

1. **Establishing Grounds for a Lawsuit:**

- **Evidence Collection:** Parents should document instances of aggressive marketing towards children—such as product placement, advertising, promotions during before-school and after-school hours, etc.
- **Health Concerns:** Establish a link between these unhealthy foods and health issues like obesity, diabetes, and other related problems in children.

2. **Seek Legal Counsel:**

- **Lawyer Specialization:** Engage a lawyer or a law firm specializing in consumer rights or class action lawsuits.
- **Initial Consultation:** Discuss the feasibility of the lawsuit, potential challenges, and the overall process.

3. **Establish a Plaintiff Group:**

- **Group Formation:** Find a group of affected parents willing to join the lawsuit, ensuring they represent a cross-section of the community for broader legitimacy.
- **Named Plaintiffs:** Among the group, select one or several individuals to be the "named plaintiffs" who will represent the group.

4. **Filing the Lawsuit:**

- **Drafting a Complaint:** With the help of legal counsel, draft a comprehensive complaint detailing allegations against the bodegas.
- **Court Submission:** Submit the complaint to a relevant court that has jurisdiction over such cases.

5. **Certification as a Class Action:**

- **Requirements:** The court will assess if the case meets class action requirements, including whether there are enough common claims among the plaintiffs.
- **Notification:** If the court certifies the case as a class action, potentially affected individuals must be notified and given an opportunity to join or opt-out.

6. **Discovery Process:**

- **Exchange of Information:** Both sides will exchange evidence. This might include marketing strategies of bodegas, sales data, health reports, and expert testimonies.

7. **Settlement or Trial:**

- **Settlement Negotiations:** Many class actions settle before reaching court. Legal counsel will negotiate terms on behalf of the plaintiff group.
- **Trial:** If no settlement is reached, the case proceeds to trial where both sides present their case, and a verdict is reached.

8. **Post-Trial Steps:**

- **Distribution of Damages:** If the verdict is in favor of the plaintiffs, damages awarded by the court are distributed among the members of the class action.
- **Appeals:** If either side disagrees with the verdict, they have the right to appeal the decision.

9. **Public Awareness and Advocacy:**

- **Media Engagement:** To strengthen their case and cause, parents should engage with media outlets to highlight the issue and gain public support.
- **Community Programs:** Advocate for educational programs in schools and communities about the dangers of unhealthy foods and the importance of balanced diets.

Conclusion

Filing a class action lawsuit against Bodegas is a complex yet vital endeavor that demands dedication, resources, and resilience. As urban parents are armed with evidence and public backing, they can confront the unethical sales practices of these establishments. Recognizing bodegas' significant influence on children's diets, it becomes imperative to use legal action as a tool to cultivate healthier urban food environments. Ultimately, the health and well-being of our children are paramount, and such steps are essential to safeguard future generations from preventable health challenges.

Final Thoughts

In "Bodegas: Urban Children Health Matters," we've journeyed through the intricate labyrinths of urban food landscapes, witnessing firsthand how small corner stores, or bodegas, influence the nutritional choices and health outcomes of urban children. These establishments, often symbolic of urban culture and convenience, paradoxically present both challenges and opportunities for improving child health. As the neon signs of bodegas glow in the twilight of busy city streets, they beckon with a siren call of readily accessible, often calorie-rich, nutrient-poor snacks. Yet, with informed community engagement and strategic intervention, they hold the potential to become epicenters of nutritional revitalization.

The health of our urban children, the future custodians of our cities, hinges on our ability to recognize and navigate these dichotomies. Addressing the bodega phenomenon isn't just about altering the food products on the shelves but about understanding deeper socio-economic structures, cultural nuances, and the pervasive power of targeted marketing. As I conclude, it becomes evident that true change will require collaboration—between store owners, communities, health professionals, and policymakers—to transform these corner stores from mere snack hubs to genuine nourishment centers.

This exploration underscores a profound truth: in the heart of the concrete jungle, every bodega, with its cacophony of choices, mirrors the broader challenges and opportunities of urban health. As I close the pages on this exploration, it is my hope that readers, empowered with knowledge and insight, will champion the cause of reimagining bodegas. In doing so, we can ensure that every urban child's health truly matters and is nurtured in the bustling aisles of these iconic city stores.

Vocabulary List

This vocabulary list provides an overview of some essential terms that might be used when discussing bodegas, children's health, and broader community and cultural influences:

1. **Bodega:** A small grocery store, especially in a Spanish-speaking neighborhood.

2. **Urban:** Related to a city or densely populated area.

3. **Dietary habits:** The habitual decisions an individual or culture makes when choosing what foods to eat.

4. **Processed foods:** Foods that have been altered from their natural state, often to make them more convenient or longer-lasting.

5. **Nutrition:** The study of food and how it affects the health of the body.

6. **Impressionable:** Easily influenced; sensitive.

7. **Parental guidance:** Advice or support given by parents to their children.

8. **External influences:** Outside factors or forces that can affect someone's decisions, behavior, or way of thinking.

9. **Community hubs:** Central places where members of a community gather or obtain services.

10. **Sugary foods:** Foods that contain a large amount of sugar, often leading to health issues if consumed in large quantities.

11. **Peer pressure:** Influence from members of one's peer group to behave in a certain way.

12. **Food desert:** An urban area in which it is difficult to buy affordable or high-quality fresh food.

13. **Wholesome:** Conducive to good health and physical well-being.

14. **Obesity:** A medical condition characterized by an excessive amount of body fat.

15. **Cultural influences:** Shared beliefs, values, and practices that influence an individual's choices and behaviors.

16. **Nutritional education:** Teaching individuals about the dietary requirements and the importance of eating healthily.

17. **Processed alternatives:** Substituted food products which are often less nutritious than whole, fresh foods.

18. **Healthy snacks:** Small portions of food that provide nutritional value and sustain energy between meals.

19. **Urban landscape:** The physical appearance of an urban area, including buildings, transportation, open spaces, and amenities.

20. **Community dynamics:** The patterns of interaction and relationships within a community.

21. **Dietary pitfalls:** Mistakes or challenges in adhering to a nutritious diet.

22. **Health implications:** Potential impacts or consequences for an individual's health.

23. **Temptations:** Desires or impulses towards something, especially when not aligned with one's long-term goals or values.

24. **Lifelong eating habits:** Dietary behaviors and choices that are formed early in life and continue throughout one's lifetime.

25. **Socioeconomic factors:** Social and economic factors that influence individuals' behaviors, attitudes, and opportunities.

26. **Nutritional understanding:** Comprehensive knowledge about the value, effects, and importance of various foods and diets.

27. **Cultural cuisine:** Traditional food from a particular culture or region.

28. **Diverse palates:** Various and distinct tastes or preferences for food.

29. **Sustainable sourcing:** Obtaining food and other goods in a way that preserves the environment and supports local producers.

30. **Dietary landscape:** The array of food choices and influences in a particular area or community.

Appendix A: Bodega Foods: What Kids Should Avoid

Here's a list of foods that kids should ideally avoid or consume in moderation when purchasing from Bodegas:

1. **Sugary Beverages:** This includes sodas, energy drinks, and excessively sweetened fruit juices or fruit drinks.

2. **Candies and Sweets:** Particularly those high in added sugars and artificial colors or flavors.

3. **Chips and Processed Snacks:** Especially those high in saturated fats, trans fats, and sodium.

4. **Processed Pastries:** Such as pre-packaged cakes, donuts, and cookies which often contain high amounts of sugar, unhealthy fats, and preservatives.

5. **Instant Noodles:** These can be high in sodium and often contain unhealthy fats.

6. **Frozen Pizzas and Microwaveable Entrees:** They're often high in sodium, preservatives, and unhealthy fats.

7. **Processed Meats:** Such as hot dogs, bacon, and pre-packaged lunch meats which can be high in sodium, preservatives, and saturated fats.

8. **Canned Foods High in Sodium or Syrups:** For
    example, canned soups with high sodium content or fruit
    cans packed in sugary syrups.

9. **Artificially Flavored and Colored Foods:** Such as
    brightly colored cereals or snacks that contain little to no
    nutritional value.

10. **Highly Caffeinated Products:** Like energy shots or
    coffee beverages with high sugar content, not suitable for
    young consumers.

11. **Chewable Tobacco or Nicotine Products:** While these
    are not foods, they can be found at some bodegas and are
    harmful and not intended for children.

12. **High Fructose Corn Syrup:** Such as candy bars, sugary
    candies, frozen desserts, breads, and energy drinks.

When shopping at bodegas or similar stores, it's essential
to read labels and make informed choices. While occasional
indulgence is okay, consistently opting for healthier
alternatives can make a big difference in overall health.

Appendix B: Healthier Bodegas Choices

Here's a list of healthier alternatives to commonly found unhealthy snacks at Bodegas:

1. **Instead of soda:** Sparkling water, unsweetened iced tea, or infused water with fresh fruit slices.

2. **Instead of candy bars and sugary candies:** Dried fruit (without added sugars), unsweetened fruit leather, or nuts.

3. **Instead of processed snack foods:** Air-popped popcorn, whole grain crackers, or roasted chickpeas.

4. **Instead of high-sugar pastries:** Whole grain muffins, oat bars, or granola bars with low added sugars.

5. **Instead of pre-packaged meals:** Pre-packaged salads with fresh vegetables, or whole grain wraps with lean protein.

6. **Instead of foods with high fructose corn syrup:** Products sweetened naturally, like with honey, maple syrup, or fruit concentrates.

7. **Instead of energy drinks:** Herbal tea, natural fruit juices (in moderation), or simply water.

8. **Instead of sugary frozen desserts:** Yogurt-based popsicles, fruit sorbets, or fresh fruit salad.

9. **Instead of processed meats:** Low-sodium turkey or chicken breast slices, hummus, or canned tuna in water.

10. **Instead of foods with trans fats:** Foods cooked in healthier oils like olive oil or foods that are baked instead of fried.

It's always a good idea to read the nutrition labels when shopping. Making informed decisions can ensure that even when shopping at a Bodega, healthier choices are within reach.

Endnotes

Borradaile, K. E., et al. (2009). The availability of snack food displays that may trigger impulse purchases in a sample of Philadelphia corner stores. *Journal of Urban Health, 86*(2), 151-159.

Coates, T. (2014). *The case for reparations.* The Atlantic.

Cummins, S., & Macintyre, S. (2006). Food environments and obesity—neighborhood or nation? *International Journal of Epidemiology, 35*(1), 100-104.

Dubois, W.E.B. (1935). *Urban reconstruction in America.* Free Press.

Feighery, Ellen C. ; Henriksen, Lisa ; Wang, Yun ; Schleicher, Nina C. ; Fortmann, Stephen P. (2006). An evaluation of four measures of adolescents' exposure to cigarette marketing in stores. *Nicotine & Tobacco Research, 8* (6), p.751-759.

Gottlieb, R., & Joshi, A. (2010). *Food justice.* MIT Press.

Grier, S. A., & Kumanyika, S. (2008). The context for choice: health implications of targeted food and beverage marketing to African Americans. *American Journal of Public Health, 98*(9), 1616-1629.

Henriksen, L ; Feighery, E C ; Schleicher, N C ; Haladjian, H H ; Fortmann, S. P. (2004). Reaching youth at the point of sale: cigarette marketing is more prevalent in stores where adolescents shop frequently. *Tobacco Control, 13* (3), p.315-318.

Henriksen, L., Feighery, E. C., Schleicher, N. C., & Fortmann, S. P. (2008). Receptivity to alcohol marketing predicts initiation of alcohol use. *Journal of Adolescent Health, 42*(1), 28-35.

Kumanyika, S.K. (2008). Environmental influences on childhood obesity: Ethnic and cultural influences in context. *Physiology & Behavior, 94*(1), 61-70.

Larson, N. I., Story, M. T., & Nelson, M. C. (2009). Neighborhood environments: disparities in access to healthy foods in the U.S. *American Journal of Preventive Medicine, 36*(1), 74-81.

Laska, M. N., Borradaile, K. E., Tester, J., Foster, G. D., & Gittelsohn, J. (2010). Healthy food availability in small urban food stores: a comparison of four US cities. *Public Health Nutrition, 13*(7), 1031-1035.

Lipperman-Kreda, S., Grube, J. W., Friend, K. B., Mair, C. (2016). Tobacco outlet density, retailer cigarette sales without ID checks and enforcement of underage tobacco laws: Associations with youths' cigarette smoking and beliefs. *Addiction (Abingdon, England), 111* (3), p.525-532

McCarthy, W. J., Mistry, R., Lu, Y., Patel, M., Zheng, H., Dietsch, B. (2009). Density of tobacco retailers near schools: Effects on tobacco use among students. *American Journal of Public Health, 99* (11), p.2006-2013.

Morland, K., Wing, S., Diez Roux, A., & Poole, C. (2002). Neighborhood characteristics associated with the location of food stores and food service places. *American Journal of Preventive Medicine, 22*(1), 23-29.

Powell, L.M., Slater, S., Mirtcheva, D., Bao, Y., & Chaloupka, F.J. (2007). Food store availability and neighborhood characteristics in the United States. *Preventive Medicine, 44*(3), 189-195.

Ravitch, D. (2010). *The death and life of the great American school system: how testing and choice are undermining education.* Basic Books.

Reynolds, K., & Cohen, N. (2016). *Beyond the kale: Urban agriculture and social justice activism in New York City.* University of Georgia Press.

Walker, R. E., Keane, C. R., & Burke, J. G. (2010). Disparities and access to healthy food in the United States: A review of food deserts literature. *Health & Place, 16*(5), 876-884.

White, M. (2011). Sisters of the soil: Urban gardening as resistance in Detroit. race/ethnicity: *Multidisciplinary Global Contexts, 5*(1), 13-28.

Williams, R. D. (2006). Race, socioeconomic status, and health the added effects of racism and discrimination. *Annals of the New York Academy of Science, 896*(1)173-183.

www.ingramcontent.com/pod-product-compliance
Lightning Source LLC
Chambersburg PA
CBHW031406250726
48656CB00002B/559